Basic Concepts of EKG

A pocket guide

A companion to
Basic concepts of EKG- A simplified approach

Harilal K Nair MSN ANP CCRN-CMC

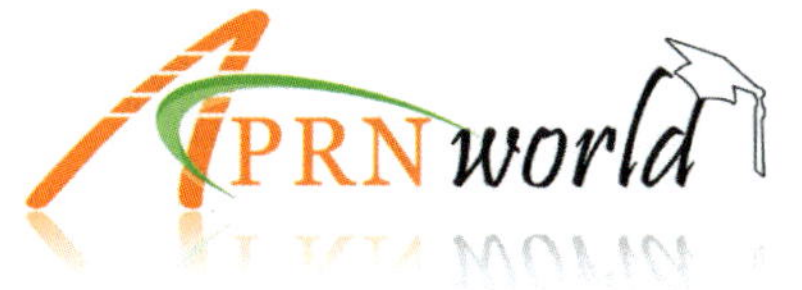

APRN World
USA

Disclaimer

This book is intended for beginners and professionals who are trying to develop better understanding of basic concept of EKG and its analysis. Therefore, this book is in no way a substitution to clinical judgment as well as established medical guidelines for actual patient care in the field. Since the modern medicine is a dynamic arena with constant addition of newer knowledge from clinical research, the author and the reviewers made genuine efforts to include most accurate and up to date information in all parts of this book. However, because of the ever-changing nature of technology and science, the author or publisher is not responsible for any inaccuracies of information especially related to drugs and devises described in this book. Since this book is not meant as a resource for active patient care, the individual learners are expected to take best efforts to identify most updated information in this regard from other available sources.

ISBN-13 978-0-9885701-4-6

Publisher Information

www.aprnworld.com

Preface

Basic concepts of EKG- A pocket guide is a supplement to the original book Basic concepts of EKG- A simplified approach. The original book was an attempt to make the complex nature of EKG analysis to a fairly simple and logical endeavor. After publishing the book, I got numerous feedbacks from my readers that the book is too big to handle in a day to day basis even though it is a great desk reference and training manual. Therefore, I thought about formatting the original book in to more concise and physically smaller in size so that everyone can use it as a pocket reference.

In the process of reducing the physical size, I tried to avoid removing any essential contents from its pure form; however, I had to compromise on certain aspects of the parent book like end of chapter review, explanation of some advanced concepts, practice tests on EKG analysis etc. I strongly believe the contents that didn't make to this pocket guide will not affect the readers since the original book was formatted as a more detailed desk reference whereas this one meant to be portable and a quick reference at bedside.

Just like the parent book, a 'rationalized approach with simplified analogy' method is used throughout this book. In order to facilitate multisensory learning of core ideas, appropriate drawings and highlights of important points are included throughout this book as its original version. I hope this will enable the students to easily skim through the chapters after their initial thorough reading.

I highly appreciate the comments and feedback I received on the original book and hope this pocket guide will also stand up to your expectation as its parent form.

Sincerely

Harilal K Nair

Table of Contents

1 Basics of EKG

Circulatory System

- Consist of a network of arteries, veins and their substructures with the heart as a central pumping organ
- In human body, there are two distinct circulatory system named **systemic circulation** and **pulmonary circulation**
- Systemic circulation carries oxygenated blood from the heart for tissue oxygenation via arteries and retrieves blood back to the heart via venous system
- Pulmonary circulation carries deoxygenated blood from the right ventricle of the heart to the pulmonary circulation and brings back oxygenated blood to the left atrium of the heart
- The human heart consists of four chambers known as *right atrium*, *right ventricle*, *left atrium*, *left ventricle* and one-way valve system to ensure unidirectional flow of blood
- Right atrium and ventricle act as the pumping system for pulmonary circulation whereas left atrium and ventricle plays the role for systemic

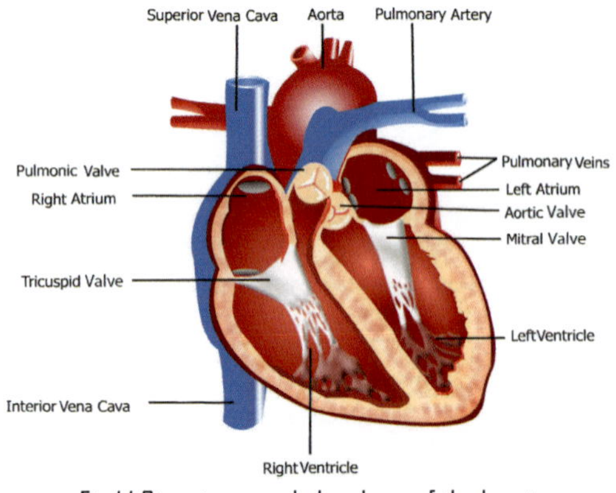

Fig 1.1 Structures and chambers of the heart

circulation

Cardiac Microstructure

- The heart wall consists of *outer pericardium*, *middle myocardium* and *inner endocardium*.
- The surface of the pericardium attached to the chest wall is called **parietal pericardium** and the one to the heart is termed as **visceral pericardium**.

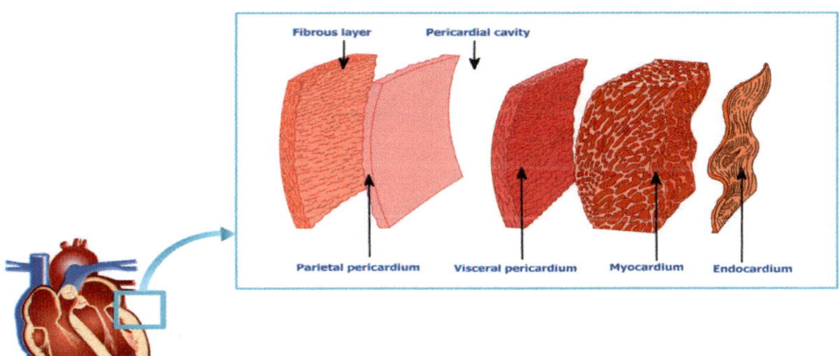

Fig 1.2 Layers of the heart wall

- **Myocardium** contains cardiac muscle cells and receive blood through epicardial coronary arteries.
- Innermost layer known as **endocardium** covers the interior of all chambers and associated structures including heart valves.

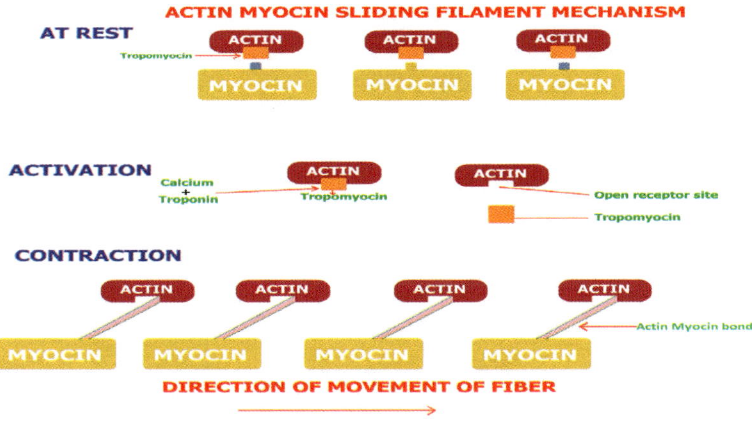

Fig 1.3 Actin Myocin sliding filament mechanism

- The building blocks of myocardium called **myocytes** consist of **sarcomere**, which is *the basic contractile units*.
- **Sarcomere** consists of thin and thick protein structures known as **actin** and **myosin filaments**.
- Movement of actin and myosin filaments through reversible binding in presence of calcium ions and ATP molecules facilitate myocardial contraction.

Cardiac Cycle

- Cardiac cycle involves a series of events happens during each heartbeat.
- It involves five phases known *isovolumetric ventricular contraction*, *ventricular ejection phase*, *isovolumetric relaxation phase*, *ventricular filling phase* and *atrial systole*. Major events during cardiac cycle are explained in Fig 1.4.

Coronary Circulation

- Epicardial coronary arteries supplies blood to the heart during *diastolic phase of the ventricle*.
- There are two main coronary artery systems known as **right** and **left coronary arteries**.

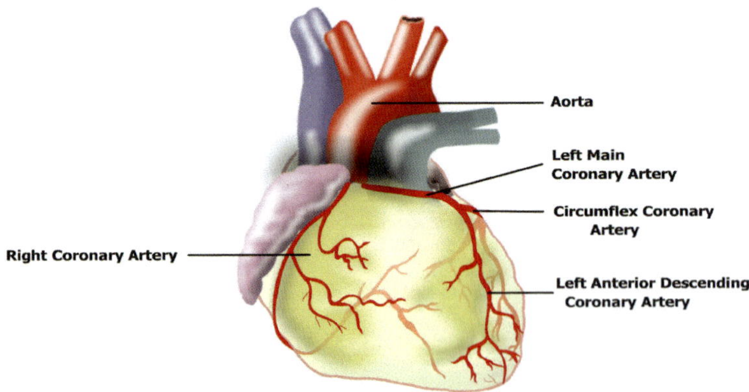

Fig 1.5 Coronary circulation

- Left coronary artery further divides into **left anterior descending artery** (LAD) and **left circumflex artery** (LCx).
- Left anterior descending artery and its branches known as Diagonal branches and septal perforators supply the anterior wall of the left ventricle and inter ventricular septum.

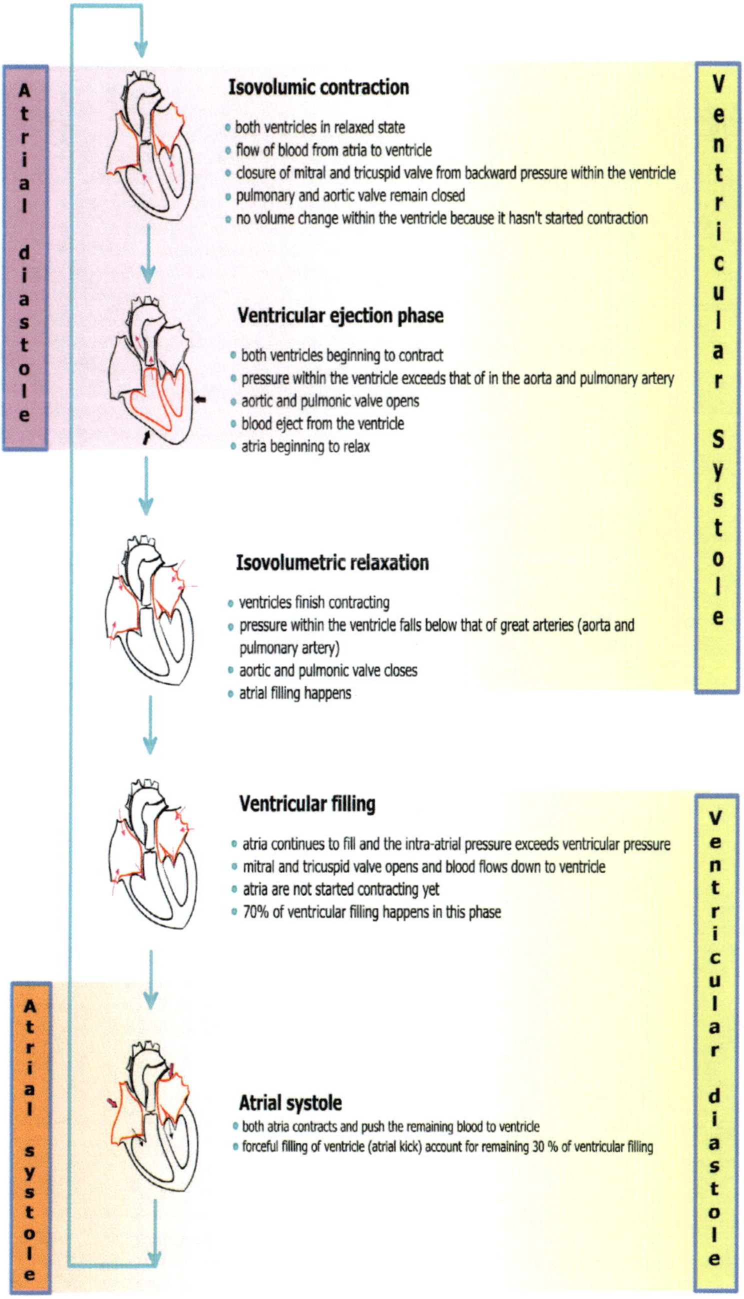

Atrial diastole

Isovolumic contraction

- both ventricles in relaxed state
- flow of blood from atria to ventricle
- closure of mitral and tricuspid valve from backward pressure within the ventricle
- pulmonary and aortic valve remain closed
- no volume change within the ventricle because it hasn't started contraction

Ventricular ejection phase

- both ventricles beginning to contract
- pressure within the ventricle exceeds that of in the aorta and pulmonary artery
- aortic and pulmonic valve opens
- blood eject from the ventricle
- atria beginning to relax

Isovolumetric relaxation

- ventricles finish contracting
- pressure within the ventricle falls below that of great arteries (aorta and pulmonary artery)
- aortic and pulmonic valve closes
- atrial filling happens

Ventricular Systole

Ventricular filling

- atria continues to fill and the intra-atrial pressure exceeds ventricular pressure
- mitral and tricuspid valve opens and blood flows down to ventricle
- atria are not started contracting yet
- 70% of ventricular filling happens in this phase

Atrial systole

Atrial systole

- both atria contracts and push the remaining blood to ventricle
- forceful filling of ventricle (atrial kick) account for remaining 30 % of ventricular filling

Ventricular diastole

Fig 1.4 Events during cardiac cycle

- Left circumflex artery and its branches known as Obtuse marginals supply the lateral and part of posterior wall of the heart.

- Right coronary artery feeds the right ventricle, inferior and some part of the posterior wall of the heart.

- Cardiac veins return all venous circulation back to the right atrium via **coronary sinus**.

Nerve Control of the Heart

- Heart is controlled by **autonomic nervous system** through its **sympathetic and parasympathetic pathways**.

- In young and healthy hearts, parasympathetic nervous system dominates the control of heart through **Vagus nerve**.

- Stimulation of vagus nerve cause parasympathetic response leading to reduction in heart rate.

Conduction System of the Heart

- Natural electrical circuit of the heart originates from **SA node** and then the impulses propagate through the atria and then to the middle **AV node**.

- AV node slows down the impulse progression to the ventricle by the phenomenon known as **AV nodal delay**.

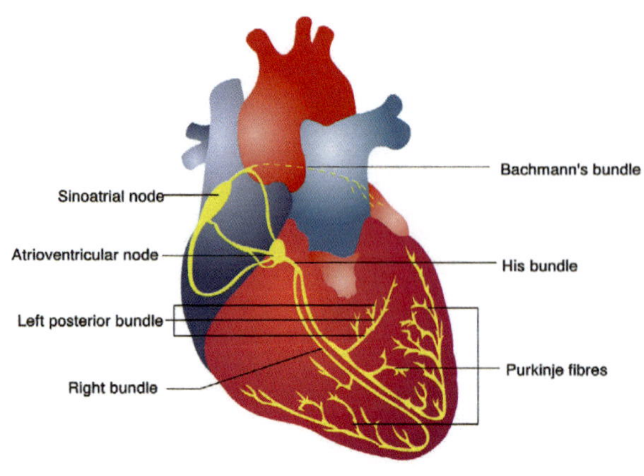

Fig 1.6 conduction system of the heart

- AV nodal delay ensures a *synchronized contraction between atria and ventricle* and is essential for adequate cardiac output.

- From the AV node, electrical impulses travel to the ventricle via **Bundle of his** and its branches known as **Purkinje fibers**.

Properties of Cardiac Cells

- Myocardial cells process unique properties known as *contractility*, *conductivity*, *automaticity* and *rhythmicity*.

- **Contractility** is the property by which cardiac tissue can contract in response to electrical stimuli.

- **Conductivity** is the ability to conduct electricity after the stimulation.

- **Automaticity** is the ability to initiate its own impulses.

Inherent Rate of Pacemaker Cells

SA node	60 to 100 bpm
AV node	40 to 60 bpm
Ventricle	20 to 40 bpm

Even though SA node is a natural pacemaker, in the event of its failure to initiate an impulse; downstream cells start generating electrical impulses in order to maintain hemodynamics. For example, the junctional rhythm which originates from AV node usually runs at 40 to 60 bpm. If the rate of junctional rhythm is more than 60 bpm it is called accelerated junctional rhythm. Similarly, during third-degree heart block or AV dissociation atrial rate will be somewhere in the order of 60 to 100 beats per minute; however ventricular rate usually is in 30 to 40 range.

Box 1.1 Inherent rate of pacemaker cells

- **Rhythmicity** is the capability of maintaining regularity of electric impulses.

Cardiac Action Potential

- During impulse transmission, myocardial cells undergo cycles of depolarization and repolarization through ion exchange.

- Cardiac action potential is the sequence of events happens in cardiac cells due to the movements of sodium, potassium and calcium ions during impulse transmission.

- There are five phases for cardiac action potential with the

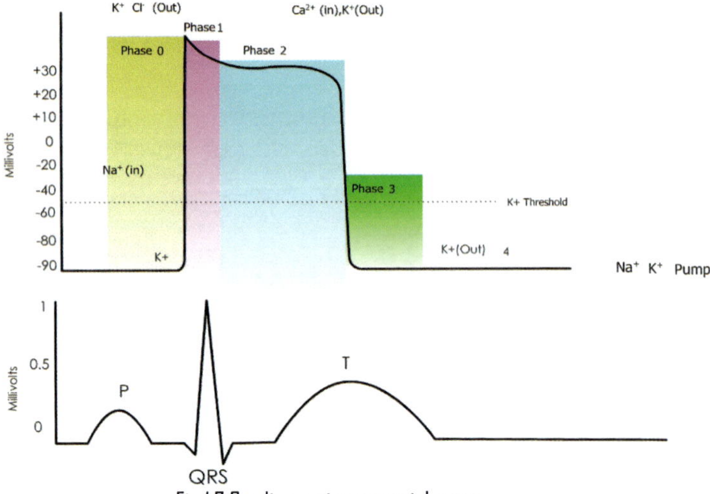

Fig 1.7 Cardiac action potential curve

characteristic ionic moments across the myocardial cell membrane.

- In **phase 0**, there is a *large influx of sodium ions into the cell* from extracellular space leading to positive polarization of intracellular space.
- During **phase 1**, *potassium ions start moving out of the cell* leading to a partial repolarization of the cell.
- In **phase 2**, *calcium ions move in through calcium channels* and *outflow of potassium ions* continues.
- Because of the bidirectional movement of positively charged calcium and potassium, a transient electrical neutrality develops as represented by the plateau phase of action potential curve.
- In **phase 3**, *potassium outflow exceeds that of calcium* leading to electrical negativity within the cell.
- Through active transport mechanisms like **sodium potassium ATPase pump** and **calcium ion pump**, excess of sodium and calcium ions that enters into the cell during initial phase of action potential are removed during **phase 4** .
- At the end of phase 4, the cardiac cells are back to their initial energy state and are ready for another action potential.
- During each cycle of cardiac action potential, there is a timeframe where the cells are not capable of responding to

another electrical stimulus called **refractory period**.

- **Absolute refractory period** is the *interval from the beginning of phase 0 of action potential to a point in phase 3*.
- During absolute refractory period, the cells are not at all capable of responding to another impulse.
- **Relative refractory period** is a time between *end of absolute*

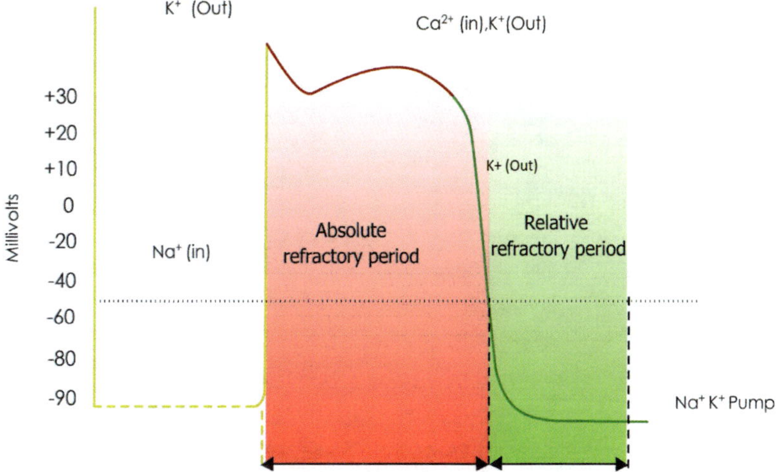

Fig 1.8 Absolute and relative refractory period

refractory period and the beginning of next action potential. During this phase a sufficiently strong stimulus can generate another action potential response.

- Abnormal stimulation during early part of relatively refractory period can cause ventricular fibrillation (As seen in R on T phenomena).

EKG Waveform

- The electrocardiogram tracing represents electrical activity of the heart.
- Since the electrical activity is synchronized with mechanical function, each part of EKG waveform represents specific mechanical function of the heart.
- The direction of complexes in an EKG wave form is determined by the direction of electrical current.
- The current flowing *towards the positive electrode generate a*

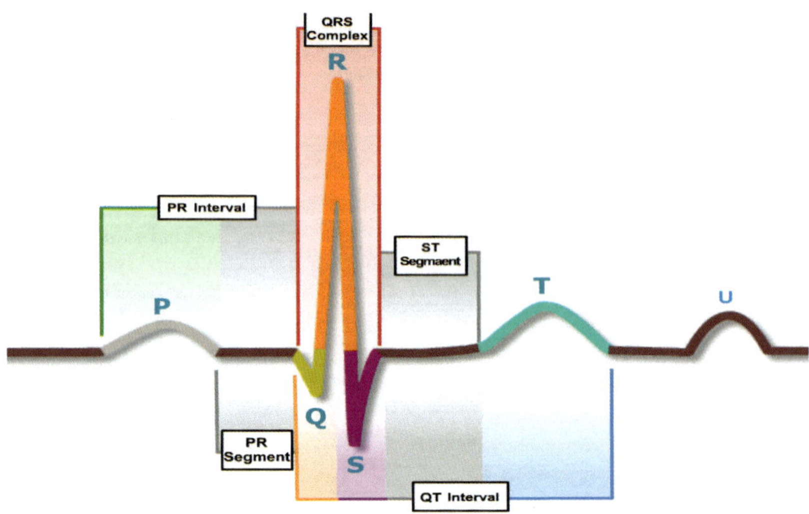

Fig 1.9 EKG waveform

positive waveform in the EKG.

- When current *flows away from the positive electrode*, *a negative waveform* is developed.
- A *biphasic or isoelectric waveform is developed when the*

Identification of Waves in EKG

P wave	*First positive deflection* in the EKG complex. It is inverted in junctional rhythms, lead aVR, V1 and in some pathologic waves. Presence of P wave determines whether the impulses are originating from the atria or somewhere else.
Q wave	*First negative deflection* in the QRS complex. A large Q wave (greater than 0.04 ms and greater than one third of R wave) represents myocardial death.
R wave	*Second positive reflection* in PQRST complex. It is usually tall in EKG leads with a positive electrode on the left side of the chest wall such as lead I, II, III, aVL, aVF, V5 and V6.
S wave	*Second negative deflection* in the PQRST complex.
T wave	*Third positive deflection* in the EKG complex. In ischemia or infarction, T waves may be inverted.
U wave	*4th positive reflection* immediately following the T wave.
J point	*The junction between end of QRS and the beginning of ST segment*. J-point is elevated in ST elevation Myocardial infarction (STEMI).

Box 1.2 Identification of waveforms in EKG

current is flowing perpendicular to the positive electrode.

- The net direction of electrical flow in the heart is directed towards the *left and downward direction* also known as *normal axis*.

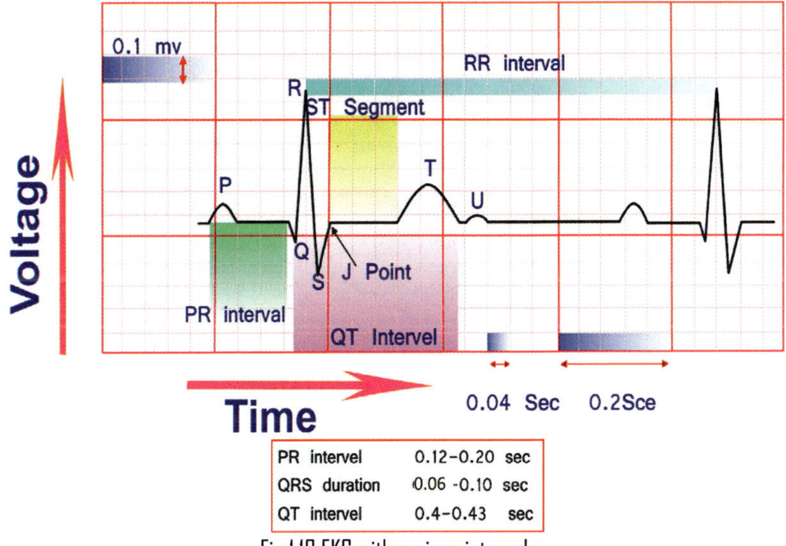

Fig 1.10 EKG with various intervals

Intervals and Measurements in EKG

Intervals and Measurement in EKG	
PR interval	*Time delay in conduction of impulse in the AV node*. It is prolonged in some types of heart block. **Normal 0.12** to **0.20 seconds**
QRS duration	*Time of ventricular repolarization* (*contraction*). This value is increased in bundle branch block and premature ventricular contraction. **Normal 0.06** to **0.10 seconds.**
QT interval	*Total time of cardiac contraction and relaxation*. Drugs like Amiodarone can elongate QT interval. **Normal 0.40** to **0.43 seconds**

Box 1.3 Intervals in EKG

- EKG is traditionally recorded on a graph paper with the *time in X axis* and *voltage in Y axis*.

- Each *small box from left-to-right indicates 0.04 seconds* and each *small box from bottom to top indicate 0.1 mV*.

Various Leads in Multichannel EKG

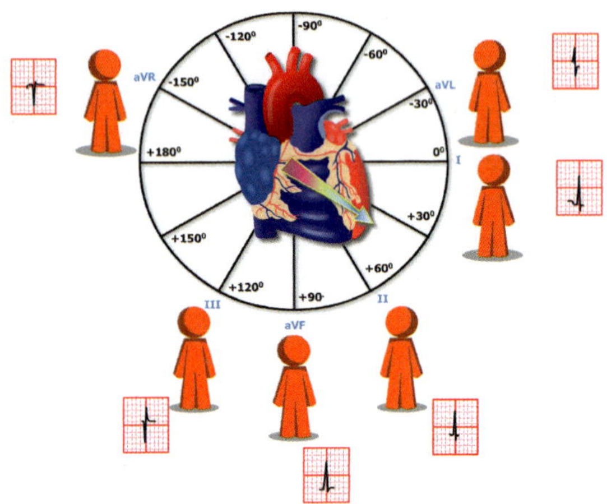

Fig 1.11 View of the heart from various vertical lead positions

- A single EKG lead represents electrical activity of the heart which is a three-dimensional structure, from one point of view.

- In order to represent electrical activity of the entire heart, multiple views from different vantage points are needed.

- In a 12 lead EKG, the electrical activity of the heart is viewed from six vertical and six

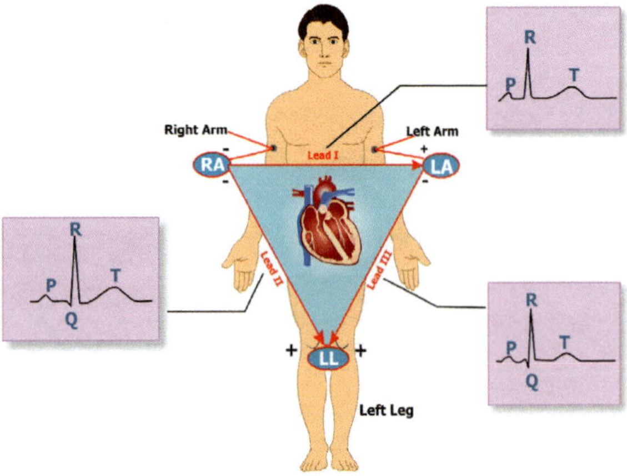

Fig 1.12 Einthoven triangle and limb leads

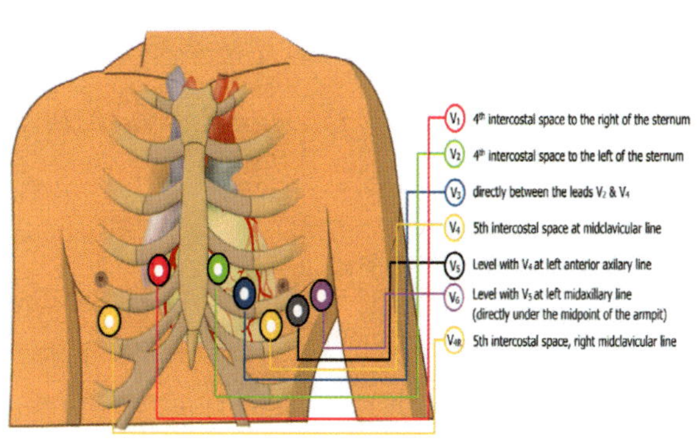

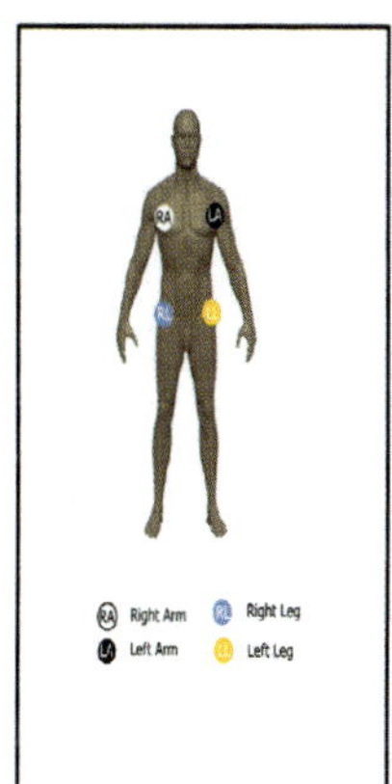

Fig 1.13 Precordial lead placement

horizontal points.

- There are two types of leads known as **unipolar** and **bipolar leads** depending on the number of electrical points attaching to the body.

Location of Precordial Leads	
V1	Fourth intercostal space on the right sternal border
V2	Fourth intercostal space on the left sternal border
V3	Between V2 and V4
V4	Fifth intercostal space in the left midclavicular line
V5	Fifth intercostal space in the left anterior axillary line
V6	Fifth intercostal space in the left mid-axillary line
V3 R	Between V1 and V4R
V4R	Fifth intercostal space on the *right midclavicular* line

Box 1.4 Location of precordial leads

- Unipolar leads have a single physical electrode attached into the body and the EKG machine calculates *electrical difference between the single available lead and an imaginary point at the center of the heart* with a zero electrical potential.

- Examples of unipolar leads are all precordial leads (V1, V2, V3 etc.) and augmented leads (aVR, aVL, aVF).

- In bipolar leads, *the electrical difference is measured between a positive and negative electrode*.

- Examples of bipolar leads are lead I, II and III.

Systematic Interpretation of EKG

- EKG should be read in a systematic and orderly fashion in

order to avoid any possibility of overlooking vital information.

- Major steps involved in interpretation of EKG are shown in the box.

Steps in EKG Interpretation

1. Determine the **rhythm** and **regularity**
2. Calculate the **rate**
3. Evaluate **P wave**
4. Calculate **PR interval**
5. Analyze **QRS complex**
6. Examine **T wave**
7. Calculate **QT interval**
8. Look for **other** characteristics

Box 1.5 Steps in EKG wave interpretation

1. Determine rhythm and regularity

- Normal EKG should have a *P wave in the beginning* , that represent atrial origin of the impulse.
- P wave should be followed by QRS complex and T wave.
- Depending on the presence or absence of P wave, rhythm can be classified into atrial or ventricular rhythm.
- If the P wave is absent, inverted or occurs after QRS complex; representing rhythm is originating from the atrio ventricular junction and is called **junctional rhythm**.
- If there is no P wave and only QRS complex, then the rhythm is ventricular in origin.

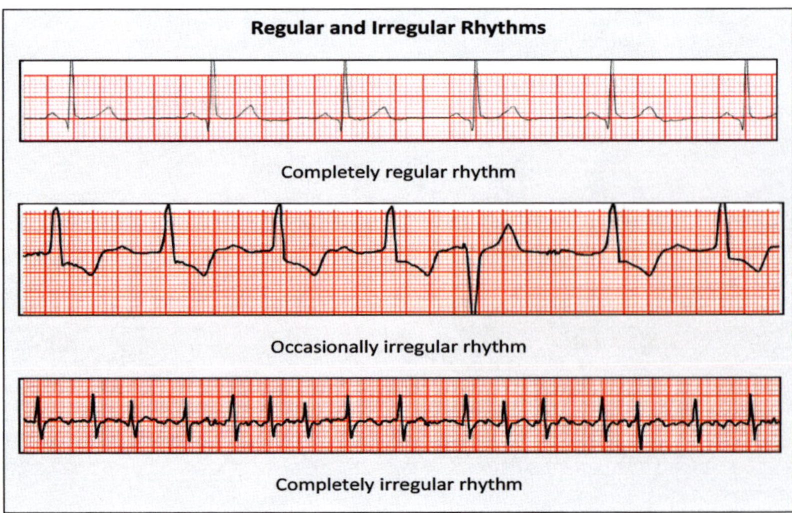

Fig 1.14 Regular and irregular rhythms

- Look for regularity of the rhythm by analyzing **P-P** and **R-R interval.** In a regular rhythm, these measurements are going to be *constant from beat to beat*.

- In some instances, the rhythm can be regular in most of the part; however, one extra beat can make the entire rhythm look irregular. Therefore, while assessing the regularity of rhythm, evaluate the entire length of available EKG tracing.

- In certain situations, these premature beats can present at regular intervals such as every other beat or every third beat (**bigeminy** and **trigeminy**) and these rhythms should be classified as *regularly irregular*.

- In completely irregular rhythms, P-P and R-R measurements will be different from beat to beat. This chaotic rhythm may have multiple P waves between each R wave as in the case of **Atrial fibrillation** and origin of R waves will be in random.

2. Calculate heart rate

- Heart rate can be calculated by various methods from an EKG

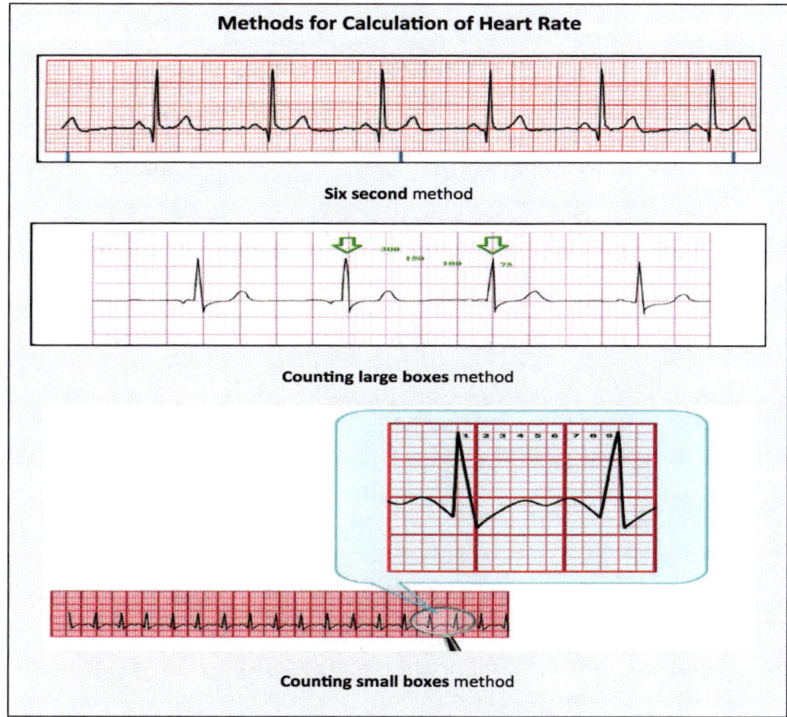

Fig 1.15 Methods for counting heart rate

strip.

- In **six second method**, *count the number of QRS complexes in a six seconds EKG strip and multiply by 10*.
- In **counting large boxes method**, *count the number of large boxes between two QRS complexes and divides into 300*.
- In **counting small box method**, *count the number of small boxes between two QRS complex and divided in to 1500*.

3. Evaluate P wave

- In normal sinus rhythm, there will be one identical P wave before each QRS complex.
- In situations where other ectopic foci within the atria produce impulses, the shape of P wave can be varying (**wandering pacemaker**).
- If the P wave appears to be *inverted*, *biphasic or following QRS*, then the **rhythm is junctional**.
- P waves are absent in pure ventricular rhythms.

4. Calculate PR interval

- **PR interval** is the time taken for the impulse to travel from atria to the ventricle.
- An **elongation of PR interval** shows additional delay for impulse to travel between the two chambers as seen in various types of heart block.
- To assess PR interval, *count the number of small boxes between the beginning of P wave to the beginning of QRS complex and multiply by 0.4*. Resulting value is the PR interval in seconds.
- PR interval *should be measured in multiple areas of the same strip* so that any irregularity in PR interval, which is the hallmark of various types of heart block can be found.

5. Analyze QRS complex

- To calculate the QRS duration, *count the number of small boxes starting from the beginning of QRS complex* (i.e. from the end of PR interval) *to the end of S wave and multiply by 0.04*. Normal QRS complex duration is **0.06 - 0.10 seconds.**

6. Evaluate T wave

- Examine the EKG for *presence of T waves after each QRS*, its *shape* (upright or inverted), *amplitude* (normally not more than 1/2 the size of R wave), *any abnormal appearance* (presence of hidden P wave within T wave) and *presence of U wave* after T waves.

7. Calculate QT interval

- QT interval represents the time duration for depolarization and repolarization of ventricles. Again, *count the number of small boxes between beginning of Q wave and end of T wave and multiply by 0.4.* Normal QT interval is between **0.36- 0.44 seconds.**

8. Other characteristics

- Look for other characteristics such as *ectopic beats*, *pauses* and *any regularity of these events*, *ST segment changes*, *dropped beats*, *presence of multiple P waves for each QRS* etc.

-

2 Understanding Arrhythmias

SA nodal rhythms

- These are cardiac rhythms originating from the **SA node**, the *natural pacemaker of the heart.*
- All of these rhythms will have the *characteristic uniform P waves before each QRS complexes*.

Mechanism Behind Origin of Arrhythmia

- Problems with Automaticity (due to suppression or acceleration of phase 4 of cardiac action potential). E.g. sinus bradycardia and sinus tachycardia.
- Impaired excitation (suppression of phase 0) E.g. Ischemic ventricular fibrillation.
- Repolarization issues (premature impulses in phase 3) E.g. Polymorphic ventricular tachycardia (Torsades de pointes) and atrial fibrillation.

Box 2.1 Mechanism behind origin of arrhythmia

Normal Sinus Rhythm

- Normal sinus rhythm occurs when an impulse originate in the SA node and then proceed to the AV node, which then progresses down to the ventricles through normal pathways resulting in a normal PQRST complex.

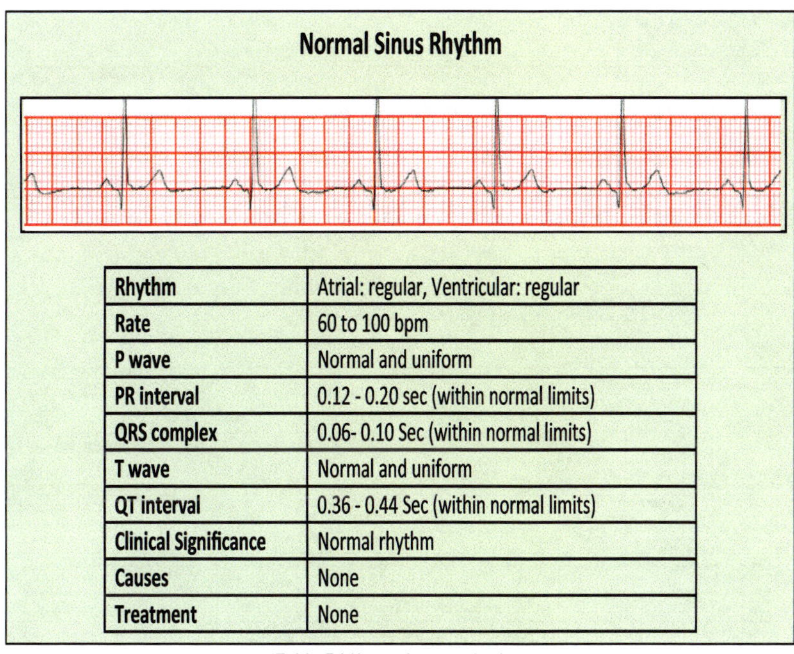

Normal Sinus Rhythm

Rhythm	Atrial: regular, Ventricular: regular
Rate	60 to 100 bpm
P wave	Normal and uniform
PR interval	0.12 - 0.20 sec (within normal limits)
QRS complex	0.06- 0.10 Sec (within normal limits)
T wave	Normal and uniform
QT interval	0.36 - 0.44 Sec (within normal limits)
Clinical Significance	Normal rhythm
Causes	None
Treatment	None

Table 2.1 Normal sinus rhythm

Sinus Arrhythmia

- Here, the heart rate stays within normal limits; however, the

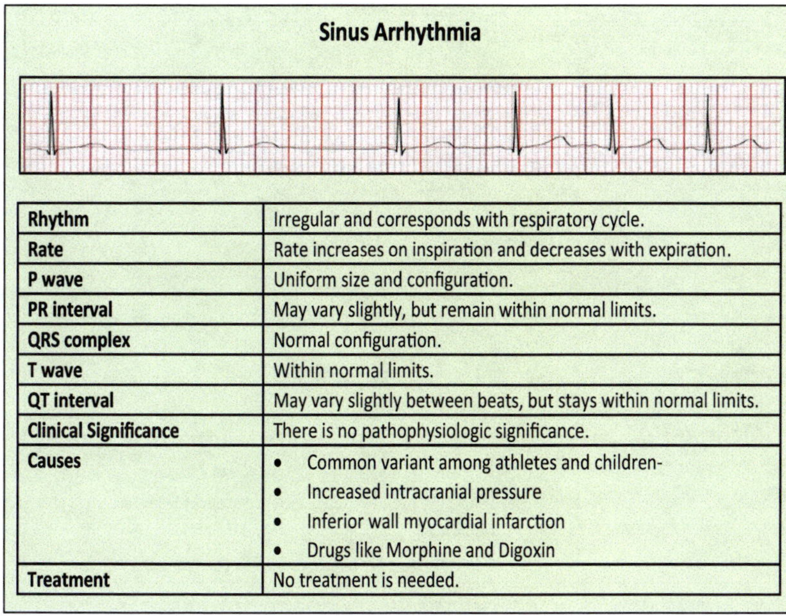

Sinus Arrhythmia

Rhythm	Irregular and corresponds with respiratory cycle.
Rate	Rate increases on inspiration and decreases with expiration.
P wave	Uniform size and configuration.
PR interval	May vary slightly, but remain within normal limits.
QRS complex	Normal configuration.
T wave	Within normal limits.
QT interval	May vary slightly between beats, but stays within normal limits.
Clinical Significance	There is no pathophysiologic significance.
Causes	• Common variant among athletes and children- • Increased intracranial pressure • Inferior wall myocardial infarction • Drugs like Morphine and Digoxin
Treatment	No treatment is needed.

Table 2.2 Sinus arrhythmia

rhythm will be irregular.

- There will be *waxing and waning of heart rate in response to respiration*.
- Sinus arrhythmia is the result of **vagal control** over the heart. It is assumed that during expiration there is a natural vagal stimulation and is responsible for slowing down of the heart rate.

Sinus Bradycardia

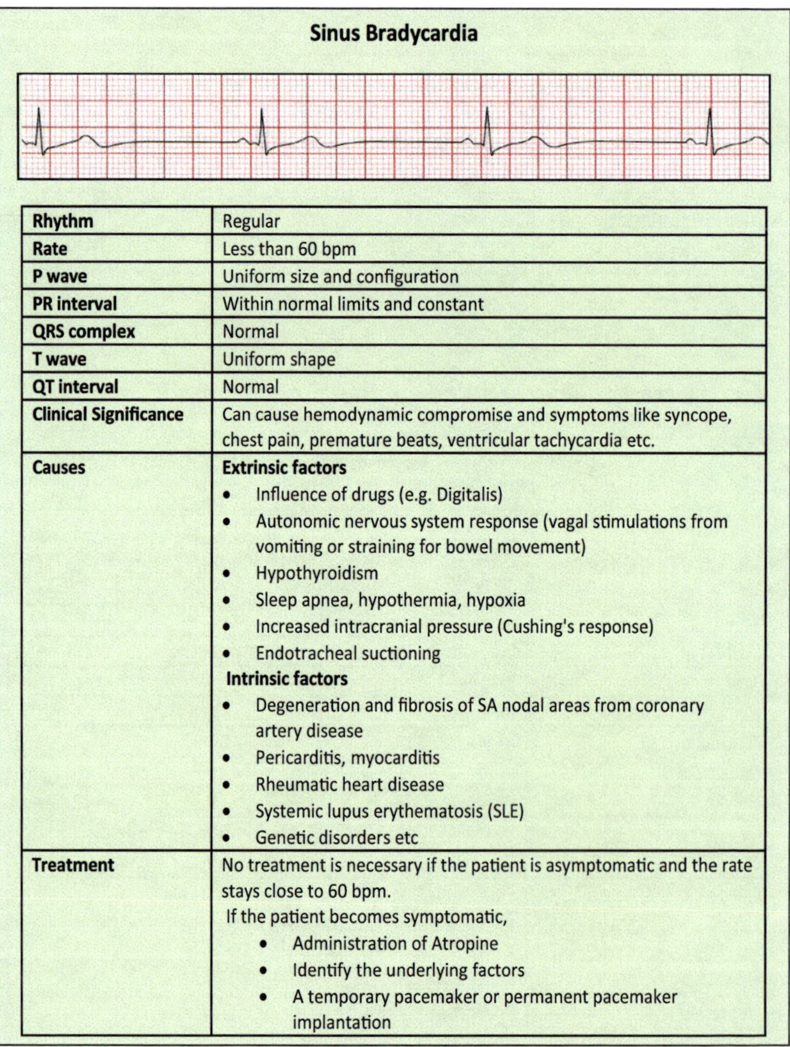

Sinus Bradycardia

Rhythm	Regular
Rate	Less than 60 bpm
P wave	Uniform size and configuration
PR interval	Within normal limits and constant
QRS complex	Normal
T wave	Uniform shape
QT interval	Normal
Clinical Significance	Can cause hemodynamic compromise and symptoms like syncope, chest pain, premature beats, ventricular tachycardia etc.
Causes	**Extrinsic factors** • Influence of drugs (e.g. Digitalis) • Autonomic nervous system response (vagal stimulations from vomiting or straining for bowel movement) • Hypothyroidism • Sleep apnea, hypothermia, hypoxia • Increased intracranial pressure (Cushing's response) • Endotracheal suctioning **Intrinsic factors** • Degeneration and fibrosis of SA nodal areas from coronary artery disease • Pericarditis, myocarditis • Rheumatic heart disease • Systemic lupus erythematosis (SLE) • Genetic disorders etc
Treatment	No treatment is necessary if the patient is asymptomatic and the rate stays close to 60 bpm. If the patient becomes symptomatic, • Administration of Atropine • Identify the underlying factors • A temporary pacemaker or permanent pacemaker implantation

Table 2.3 Sinus Bradycardia

- This rhythm is characterized by *sinus rhythm with heart rate below 60 bpm*.

Sinus Tachycardia

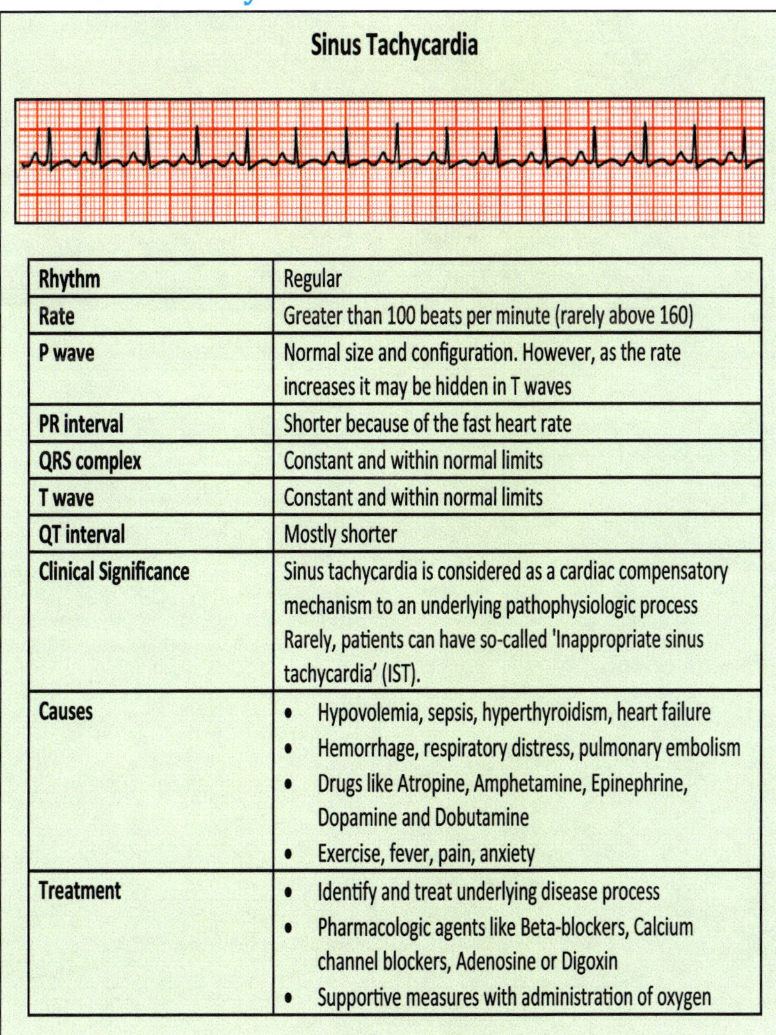

Sinus Tachycardia

Rhythm	Regular
Rate	Greater than 100 beats per minute (rarely above 160)
P wave	Normal size and configuration. However, as the rate increases it may be hidden in T waves
PR interval	Shorter because of the fast heart rate
QRS complex	Constant and within normal limits
T wave	Constant and within normal limits
QT interval	Mostly shorter
Clinical Significance	Sinus tachycardia is considered as a cardiac compensatory mechanism to an underlying pathophysiologic process Rarely, patients can have so-called 'Inappropriate sinus tachycardia' (IST).
Causes	• Hypovolemia, sepsis, hyperthyroidism, heart failure • Hemorrhage, respiratory distress, pulmonary embolism • Drugs like Atropine, Amphetamine, Epinephrine, Dopamine and Dobutamine • Exercise, fever, pain, anxiety
Treatment	• Identify and treat underlying disease process • Pharmacologic agents like Beta-blockers, Calcium channel blockers, Adenosine or Digoxin • Supportive measures with administration of oxygen

Table 2.4 Sinus tachycardia

- Sinus tachycardia involves *accelerated firing of SA node with a rate greater than 100* beats per minute.

Sinus Arrest

- A normal sinus rhythm is *interrupted by prolonged failure of SA node to initiate an impulse* resulting in complete missing of

Sinus Arrest

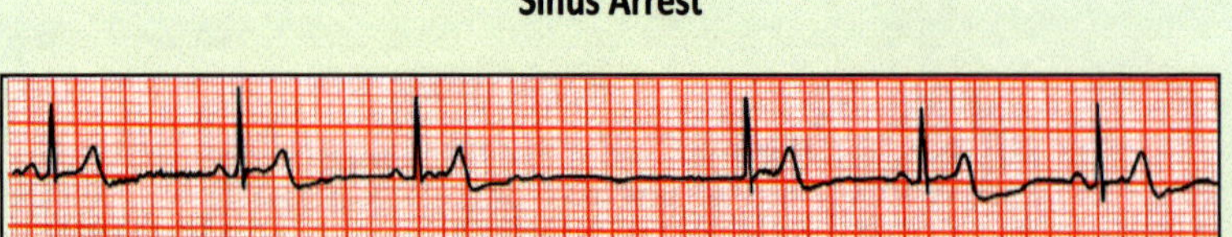

Rhythm	Regular except in missing complex (pause)
Rate	Usually within normal limits; however, length and frequency of pauses may lead to bradycardia
P wave	Normal except during pause with missing PQRST complex. The P wave may retain its uniform shape as before, depending on whether SA node or other ectopic pacemakers regain function immediately after the pause.
PR interval	Within normal limits; however, may be different in following EKG complex depends on the origin of impulse.
QRS complex	One complete QRS complex will be absent during the pause. Following QRS may assume its shape depending on whether it is SA nodal rhythm or escape beat.
T wave	Normal except during Sinus arrest where there is no T wave. Again, depending on the site of origin of impulse, it may be normal or abnormal in the following beats
QT interval	Same as in T wave; absent during pause and normal or abnormal in the following beats
Clinical Significance	Patients are asymptomatic when the length of pause is shorter; however, longer pause can create hemodynamic compromise and may need intervention.
Causes	• Ischemia affecting SA node (inferior wall MI) • Cardiomyopathy and hypertensive heart disease • Myocarditis, Sick sinus syndrome • Effect of SA nodal blocking drugs (e.g. Beta blockers, Digoxin, Amiodarone, Non-dihydropyridine calcium channel blockers) • Excessive vagal tone.
Treatment	Depends on the underlying reasons and presenting symptoms. Treatment options are same as that of sinus bradycardia

Table 2.5 Sinus arrest

PQRST complex.

Sinus Exit Block

- Here, sinus node fires impulse; however, *it doesn't generate a subsequent QRST complex because of the lack of conduction down the pathway*.
- Unlike in sinus arrest, this is a *conduction disturbance rather*

than problem with cell automaticity.

Sinus Exit Block

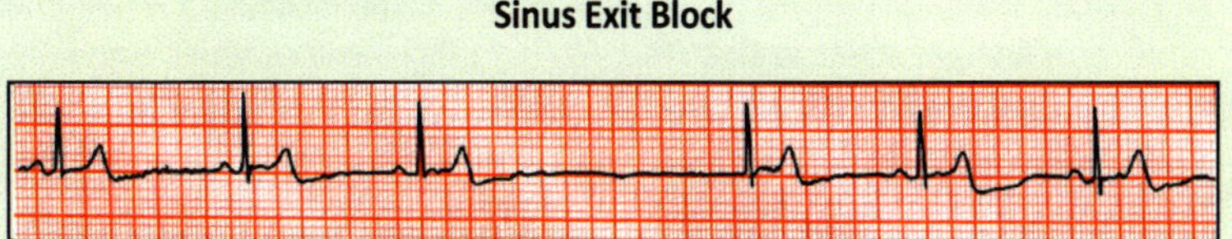

Rhythm	Regular except during pause
Rate	Usually within normal limits; however, bradycardia if length of pause is long. Length of pause is a multiplier of R-R interval
P wave	Periodically absent during pause, otherwise normal
PR interval	Normal except during the pause
QRS complex	Within normal limits; missing during pause
T wave	Absent during the pause
Clinical Significance	If the length of pause is longer, it may cause hemodynamic compromise or subjective symptoms
Causes	• Coronary artery disease and acute inferior wall myocardial infarction • Sinus node disease and Sick sinus syndrome • Myocarditis and cardiomyopathy • Drugs (e.g. Beta blockers, Calcium channel blockers, Digoxin)
Treatment	Treat as if sinus bradycardia

Table 2.6 Sinus exit block

Sick Sinus Syndrome (SSS)

Sick sinus syndrome (SSS) is a clinical condition with sickness of the natural pacemaker of the heart. It is also known as **Stokes-Adams attack**. Failure of SA node to generate impulses leads to activation of ectopic pacemakers within the atria and resultant tachyarrhythmia mostly in the form of atrial fibrillation or flutter.

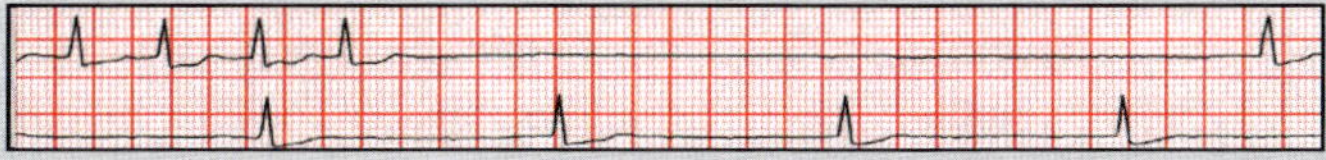

The automaticity of pacemaker cells diminishes after they have been excited with an impulse at a higher frequency such as in atrial fibrillation and is known as **override suppression phenomena**. Even after the ectopic foci stop firing, SA node cells remain dormant for little longer. The time taken for SA node to reclaim its pacemaker function after the end of tachyarrhythmia is called **sinus node recovery time**.

In patients with sick sinus syndrome, this recovery time maybe longer than usual. This leads to creation of a long pause in the EKG. Absence of cardiac output during this time can cause clinical symptoms. If the period of asystole is significantly long, patients can have loss of consciousness. Since the heart rhythm varies between tachycardia and bradycardia, it is also called '**tachy-brady syndrome**'.

Sick sinus syndrome is caused by factors leading to either degeneration or trauma to the SA node like atherosclerotic heart disease, cardiomyopathy, hypertension, pericarditis, rheumatic heart disease, valve surgery etc. It can also be precipitated by cardiac drugs like Beta-blockers, Calcium channel blockers and Digoxin. These patients may require permanent pacemaker to treat bradycardia and rate control agents like Beta-blockers and Calcium channel blocker for tachycardia.

Box 2.2 Sick sinus syndrome

- There may be one or more P waves get blocked, leading to a pause in the rhythm.
- The most distinguishable character between sinus exit block and sinus arrest is that the *pause will be a multiplier of R-R interval*.

Atrial Dysrhythmia

- These rhythms originate from *ectopic foci within the atria other than SA node*.
- They carry P wave, which may get buried in the neighboring QRS if rate is high and has a narrow QRS complex except in selected situations with presence of aberrant conduction systems.

Premature Atrial Complexes (PAC)

- PAC's are formed when an ectopic focus within the atria generate a premature impulse, which either conducted down through the AV node or die down within atria itself.

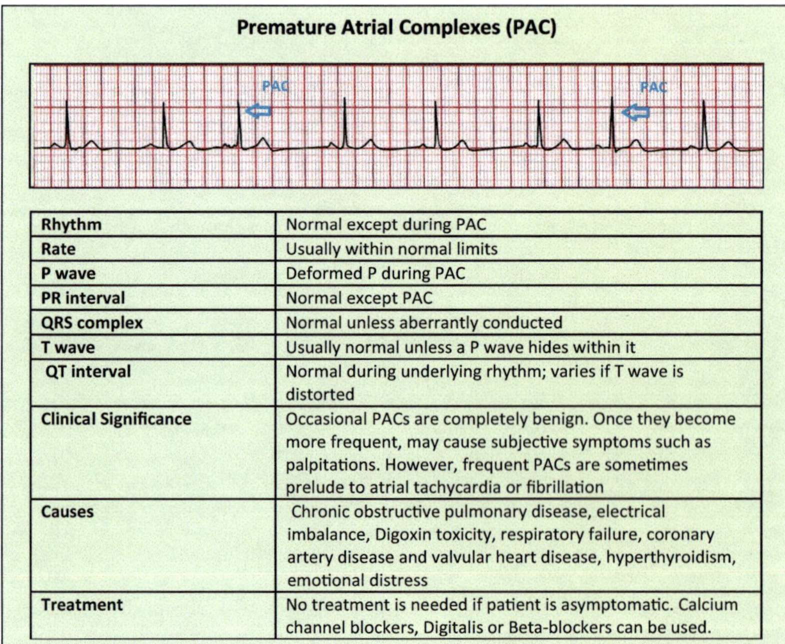

Premature Atrial Complexes (PAC)

Rhythm	Normal except during PAC
Rate	Usually within normal limits
P wave	Deformed P during PAC
PR interval	Normal except PAC
QRS complex	Normal unless aberrantly conducted
T wave	Usually normal unless a P wave hides within it
QT interval	Normal during underlying rhythm; varies if T wave is distorted
Clinical Significance	Occasional PACs are completely benign. Once they become more frequent, may cause subjective symptoms such as palpitations. However, frequent PACs are sometimes prelude to atrial tachycardia or fibrillation
Causes	Chronic obstructive pulmonary disease, electrical imbalance, Digoxin toxicity, respiratory failure, coronary artery disease and valvular heart disease, hyperthyroidism, emotional distress
Treatment	No treatment is needed if patient is asymptomatic. Calcium channel blockers, Digitalis or Beta-blockers can be used.

Table 2.7 Premature atrial complex

Atrial Tachycardia

- Also known as **Supraventricular tachycardia** (SVT) because all of them originate above the level of ventricle.
- Common forms of atrial tachycardia are **Paroxysmal atrial tachycardia** (PAT) and **Multifocal atrial tachycardia** (MAT) or so-called '**wandering pacemaker**'.
- These rhythms are characterized by an *atrial rate of 150 to 250 bpm*.
- Physiologically, these accelerated atrial rhythms diminish '*atrial kick*', which is responsible for approximately 30% of ventricular filling. This may eventually affect cardiac output.

Paroxysmal Atrial Tachycardia (PAT)

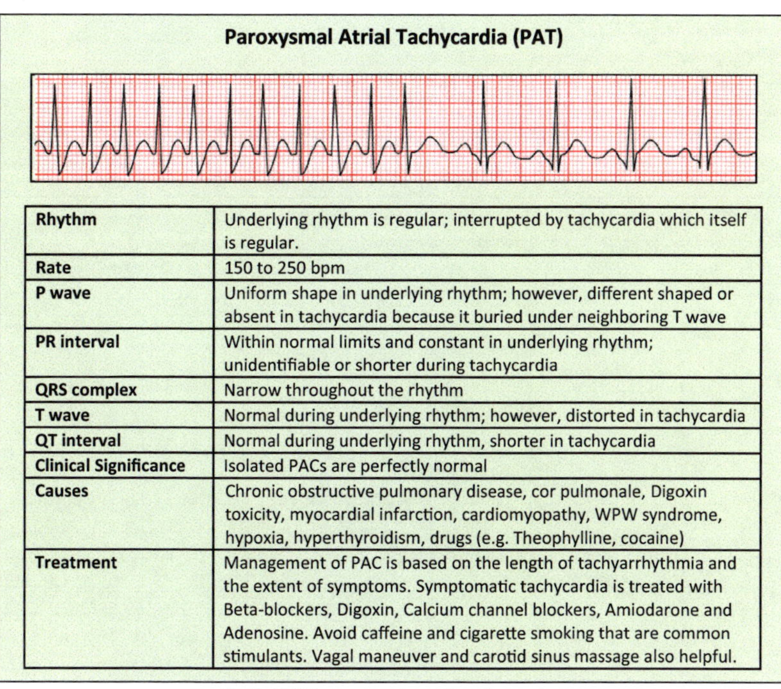

Paroxysmal Atrial Tachycardia (PAT)

Rhythm	Underlying rhythm is regular; interrupted by tachycardia which itself is regular.
Rate	150 to 250 bpm
P wave	Uniform shape in underlying rhythm; however, different shaped or absent in tachycardia because it buried under neighboring T wave
PR interval	Within normal limits and constant in underlying rhythm; unidentifiable or shorter during tachycardia
QRS complex	Narrow throughout the rhythm
T wave	Normal during underlying rhythm; however, distorted in tachycardia
QT interval	Normal during underlying rhythm, shorter in tachycardia
Clinical Significance	Isolated PACs are perfectly normal
Causes	Chronic obstructive pulmonary disease, cor pulmonale, Digoxin toxicity, myocardial infarction, cardiomyopathy, WPW syndrome, hypoxia, hyperthyroidism, drugs (e.g. Theophylline, cocaine)
Treatment	Management of PAC is based on the length of tachyarrhythmia and the extent of symptoms. Symptomatic tachycardia is treated with Beta-blockers, Digoxin, Calcium channel blockers, Amiodarone and Adenosine. Avoid caffeine and cigarette smoking that are common stimulants. Vagal maneuver and carotid sinus massage also helpful.

Table 2.8 Paroxysmal atrial tachycardia

- Characterized by *sudden onset of three or more beats of narrow complex tachycardia*; *usually originate with a premature atrial contraction*.
- They last only for a short duration and is therefore called

'paroxysmal'.

- It resembles sinus tachycardia; however, *the characteristic initiating PAC is visible* here.

Multifocal Atrial Tachycardia (MAT)

- Also known as **wandering pacemaker**, characterized by *more than one morphology of P waves*.

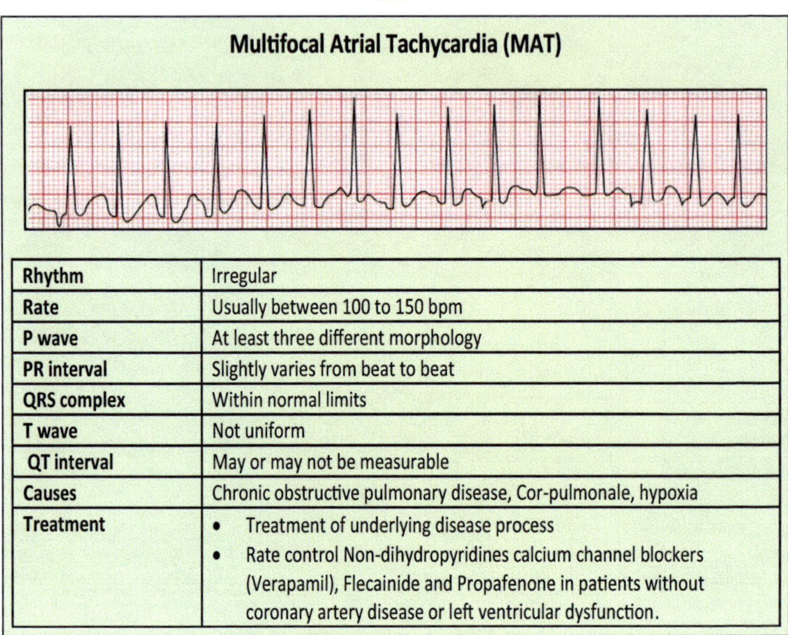

Multifocal Atrial Tachycardia (MAT)

Rhythm	Irregular
Rate	Usually between 100 to 150 bpm
P wave	At least three different morphology
PR interval	Slightly varies from beat to beat
QRS complex	Within normal limits
T wave	Not uniform
QT interval	May or may not be measurable
Causes	Chronic obstructive pulmonary disease, Cor-pulmonale, hypoxia
Treatment	• Treatment of underlying disease process • Rate control Non-dihydropyridines calcium channel blockers (Verapamil), Flecainide and Propafenone in patients without coronary artery disease or left ventricular dysfunction.

Table 2.9 Multifocal atrial tachycardia

- During this event, *impulses are originating from multiple atrial ectopic foci* and hence, different shape for P wave.
- Usually *more than three identifiable types of P waves* can be seen.

Atrial Flutter

- A form of supraventricular tachycardia with an *atrial rate of 250 to 400 bpm*.
- An aberrant pathway causing re-entry of the impulse usually generates this type of rhythm, leading to *recurrent atrial depolarization*.

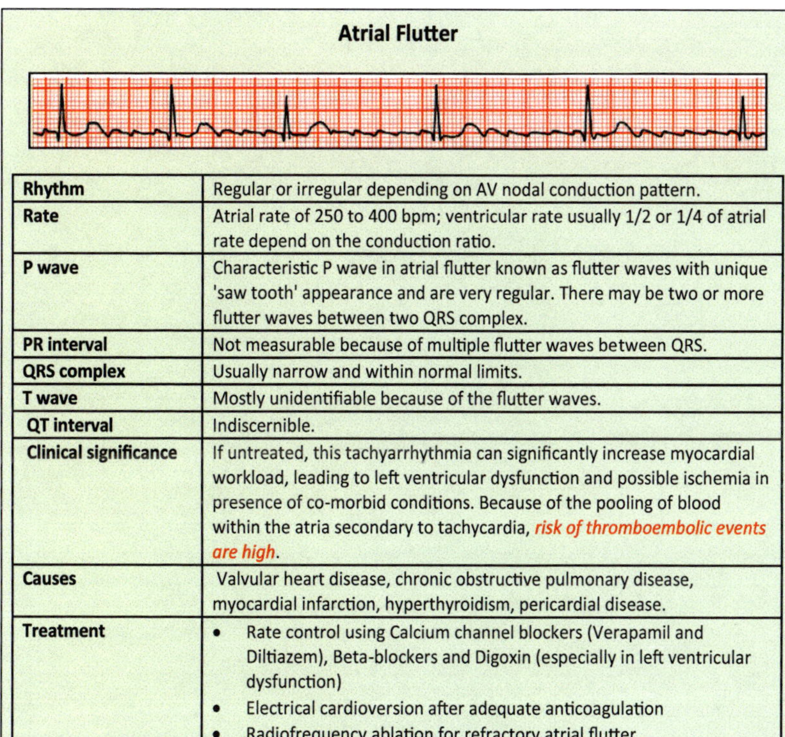

Atrial Flutter

Rhythm	Regular or irregular depending on AV nodal conduction pattern.
Rate	Atrial rate of 250 to 400 bpm; ventricular rate usually 1/2 or 1/4 of atrial rate depend on the conduction ratio.
P wave	Characteristic P wave in atrial flutter known as flutter waves with unique 'saw tooth' appearance and are very regular. There may be two or more flutter waves between two QRS complex.
PR interval	Not measurable because of multiple flutter waves between QRS.
QRS complex	Usually narrow and within normal limits.
T wave	Mostly unidentifiable because of the flutter waves.
QT interval	Indiscernible.
Clinical significance	If untreated, this tachyarrhythmia can significantly increase myocardial workload, leading to left ventricular dysfunction and possible ischemia in presence of co-morbid conditions. Because of the pooling of blood within the atria secondary to tachycardia, *risk of thromboembolic events are high*.
Causes	Valvular heart disease, chronic obstructive pulmonary disease, myocardial infarction, hyperthyroidism, pericardial disease.
Treatment	• Rate control using Calcium channel blockers (Verapamil and Diltiazem), Beta-blockers and Digoxin (especially in left ventricular dysfunction) • Electrical cardioversion after adequate anticoagulation • Radiofrequency ablation for refractory atrial flutter

Table 2.10 Atrial flutter

- The most characteristic pattern of atrial flutter is '*saw tooth*' shaped P waves called **flutter waves**.
- Because of the inherent safety mechanism within the AV node, many of these impulses terminated at the level of AV node leading to 2:1 or 4:1 conduction ratio in the ventricle.
- Even if there is 2:1 block exists, ventricles may be firing up to 150 bpm and can create serious hemodynamic compromise.

Atrial Fibrillation

- Most common and sustained atrial arrhythmia characterized by *rapid, disorganized and irregular atrial activation, most likely from multiple ectopic foci*.
- This multi center stimulation of atria results in disorganized depolarization and practically a 'trembling' or 'vibrating' movement of the atria.
- Here, AV node acts as a natural protective mechanism for

the ventricles. It blocks most of these erratic impulses and only allows smaller number of them to conduct down to the ventricles; leading to *controlled ventricular response* (CVR).

- In some instances, AV node allows most of these fibrillatory waves to pass down to ventricles leading to *rapid ventricular response* (RVR)

- There are uneven baseline fibrillatory waves and irregular QRS complexes seen in EKG.

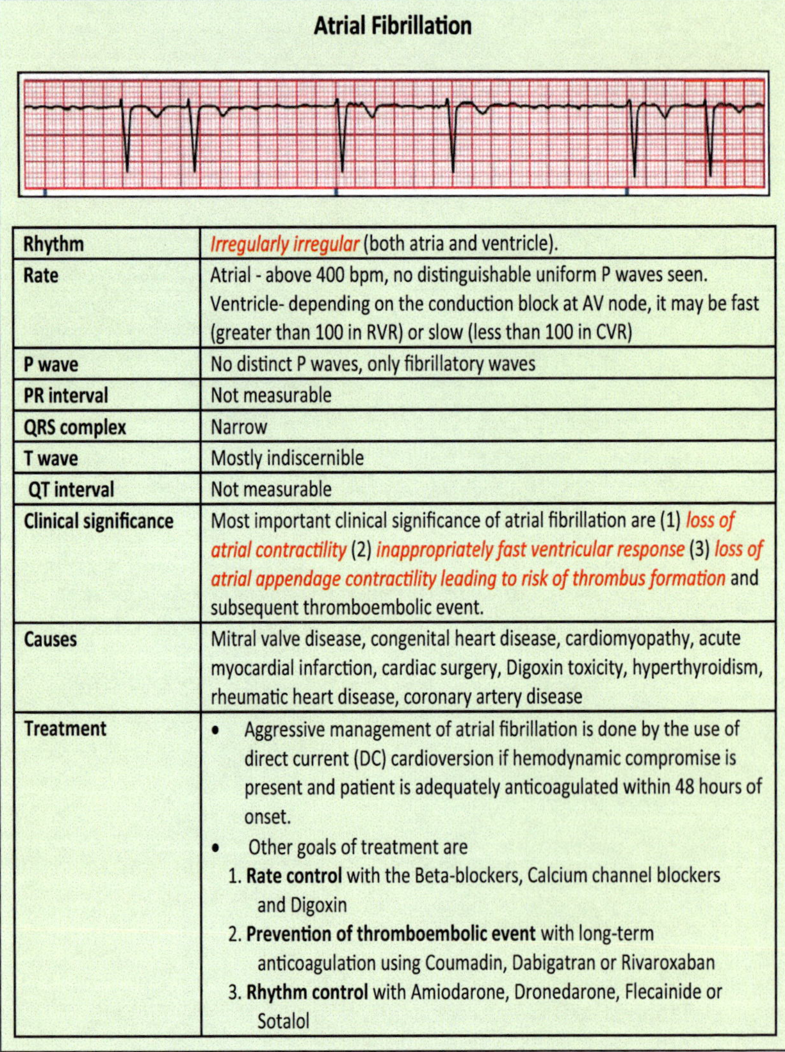

Atrial Fibrillation

Rhythm	*Irregularly irregular* (both atria and ventricle).
Rate	Atrial - above 400 bpm, no distinguishable uniform P waves seen. Ventricle- depending on the conduction block at AV node, it may be fast (greater than 100 in RVR) or slow (less than 100 in CVR)
P wave	No distinct P waves, only fibrillatory waves
PR interval	Not measurable
QRS complex	Narrow
T wave	Mostly indiscernible
QT interval	Not measurable
Clinical significance	Most important clinical significance of atrial fibrillation are (1) *loss of atrial contractility* (2) *inappropriately fast ventricular response* (3) *loss of atrial appendage contractility leading to risk of thrombus formation* and subsequent thromboembolic event.
Causes	Mitral valve disease, congenital heart disease, cardiomyopathy, acute myocardial infarction, cardiac surgery, Digoxin toxicity, hyperthyroidism, rheumatic heart disease, coronary artery disease
Treatment	• Aggressive management of atrial fibrillation is done by the use of direct current (DC) cardioversion if hemodynamic compromise is present and patient is adequately anticoagulated within 48 hours of onset. • Other goals of treatment are 1. **Rate control** with the Beta-blockers, Calcium channel blockers and Digoxin 2. **Prevention of thromboembolic event** with long-term anticoagulation using Coumadin, Dabigatran or Rivaroxaban 3. **Rhythm control** with Amiodarone, Dronedarone, Flecainide or Sotalol

Table 2.11 Atrial fibrillation

Ashman's Phenomenon

This is a *form of aberrant conduction commonly associated with atrial fibrillation*. A premature atrial impulse forms after a long RR interval will be conducted aberrantly (through an alternate pathway within the ventricle) because one bundle branch is not completely recovered from the previous impulse. In general, Right bundle has a slower refractory period than that of Left bundle and therefore the *resulting impulse has a Right bundle branch block configuration* of **rsR'** pattern. It usually results in a small number of wide complex beats on an otherwise narrow complex rhythm.

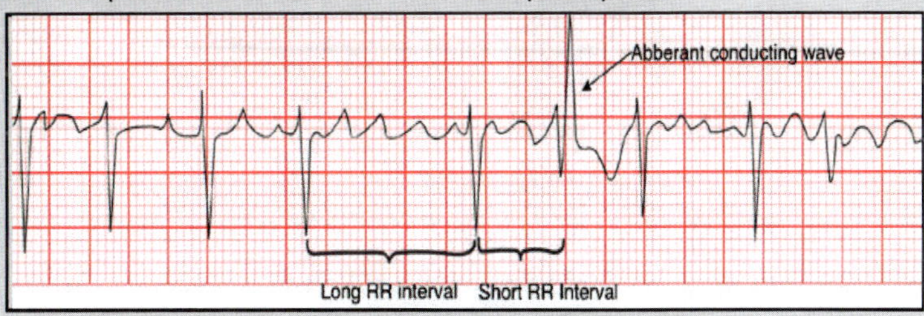

There is so called **Long Short rule for Ashman Phenomenon** as follows. *The earlier in the cycle the PAC occurs and the longer the previous cycle*, *more likely the PAC will be conducted through aberrant pathway within the ventricle*. Clinical significance of Ashman' phenomena is that it should be differentiated from serious preexcitation conditions such as WPW syndrome.

Box 2.3 Ashman's phenomenon

- Depending on the duration of atrial fibrillation, it can be classified into
- 1. **Paroxismal atrial fibrillation** (recurrent episodes that self terminate in less than seven days)
- 2. **Persistent atrial fibrillation** (recurrent episodes last more than seven days)
- 3. **Permanent or chronic atrial fibrillation** (ongoing long-term episode)

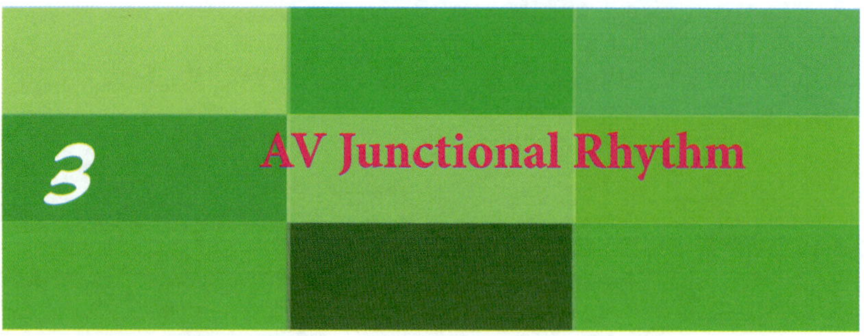

3 AV Junctional Rhythm

- The junctional rhythm or junctional escape beat is a *pacemaker impulse originating within the atrioventricular node*.
- Because of the inherent automaticity, the rate at which the AV node produces impulse is lower than that of the SA node and is about **40 to 60 beats per minute**.
- Junctional rhythms are usually seen when there are *no electrical impulses coming down from the SA node or anywhere else from the atria*.
- Since the AV node is sitting in between the atria and the ventricle, electrical impulses originating at the AV node can travel *forward to the ventricles (ante grade conduction) or backward up to the atria (retrograde conduction)*.

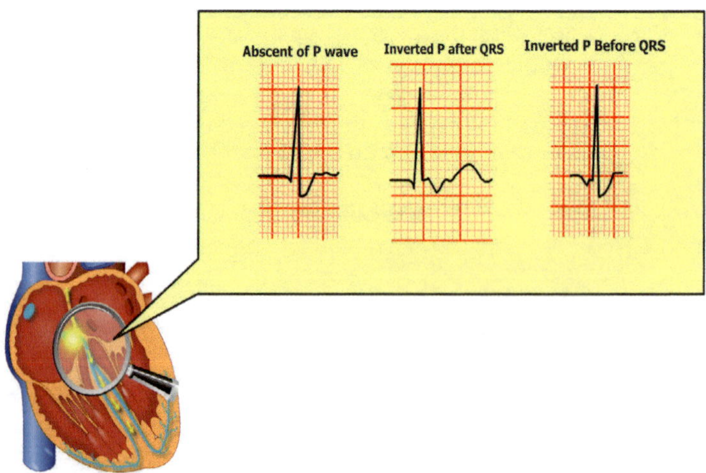

Fig 3.1 Junctional rhythm with three different morphology of P waves

Premature Junctional Contraction (PJC)

- These rhythms are originating from an *ectopic focus within the AV junction*.

- This beat occurs before a normal sinus rhythm and it depolarizes the **atria** *retrograde* (backwards) and the **ventricle** *antegrade* (forward), producing an *inverted P wave and a normal QRS complex*.

Depending on the location of impulse origin within the AV node, the *P wave can be inverted*, *absent* or *trailing.*

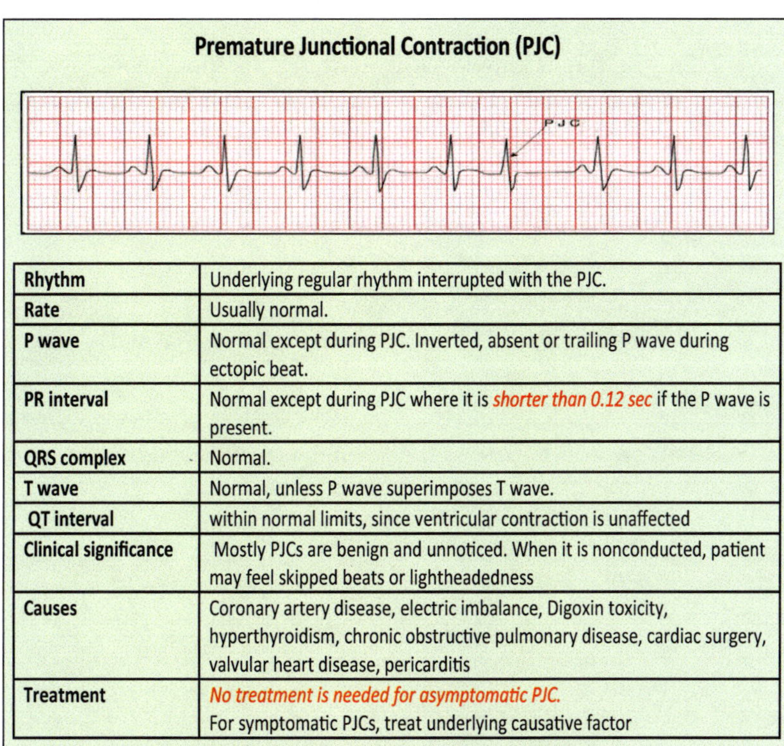

Premature Junctional Contraction (PJC)

Rhythm	Underlying regular rhythm interrupted with the PJC.
Rate	Usually normal.
P wave	Normal except during PJC. Inverted, absent or trailing P wave during ectopic beat.
PR interval	Normal except during PJC where it is *shorter than 0.12 sec* if the P wave is present.
QRS complex	Normal.
T wave	Normal, unless P wave superimposes T wave.
QT interval	within normal limits, since ventricular contraction is unaffected
Clinical significance	Mostly PJCs are benign and unnoticed. When it is nonconducted, patient may feel skipped beats or lightheadedness
Causes	Coronary artery disease, electric imbalance, Digoxin toxicity, hyperthyroidism, chronic obstructive pulmonary disease, cardiac surgery, valvular heart disease, pericarditis
Treatment	*No treatment is needed for asymptomatic PJC.* For symptomatic PJCs, treat underlying causative factor

Table 3.1 Premature junctional contraction

Junctional Rhythm

- Also known as the **Junctional escape rhythm** with a heart rate of **40** to **60 bpm** with all the characteristics of junctional type P waves throughout the rhythm.

- Common causes for junctional rhythms are *increased vagal tone*, *toxicity with Beta and Calcium blockers*, *coronary artery disease*, *degenerative changes in SA node* etc.

Junctional Bradycardia

- Here, the rate of cardiac contraction will be *less than 40 bpm*.
- If there is hemodynamic compromise, aggressive management with *transcutaneous* or *intravenous pacemaker*
- *Atropine* may also be useful in this setting.

Accelerated Junctional Rhythm

- This rhythm is known as 'accelerated' because it fires impulses *above the inherent rate of junctional tissue*, which is 40 to 60 bpm.
- Similar to other junctional impulses, they are produced as a *coping mechanism of heart* when the atrial impulses terminate.
- Along with other characteristics of the junctional rhythm, the rate will be between *60 to 100 bpm*.

Junctional Tachycardia

- This type of rhythm happens when an *ectopic junctional focus starts firing at rate above 100 bpm*.

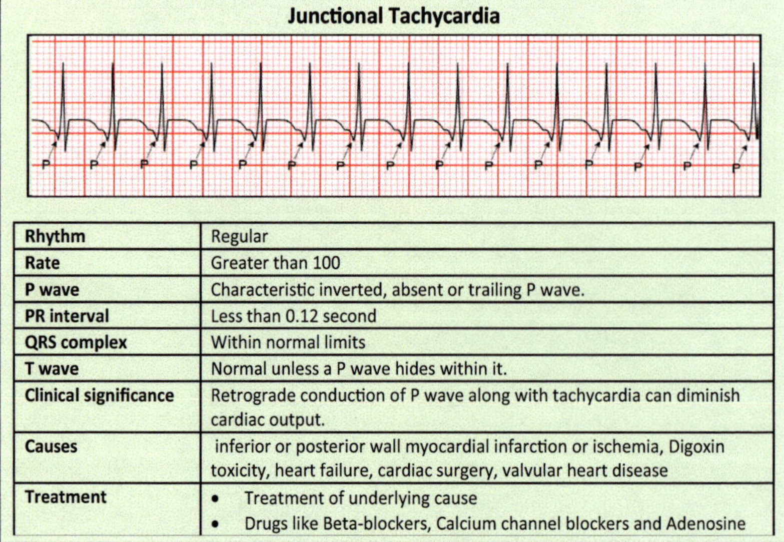
Junctional Tachycardia

Rhythm	Regular
Rate	Greater than 100
P wave	Characteristic inverted, absent or trailing P wave.
PR interval	Less than 0.12 second
QRS complex	Within normal limits
T wave	Normal unless a P wave hides within it.
Clinical significance	Retrograde conduction of P wave along with tachycardia can diminish cardiac output.
Causes	inferior or posterior wall myocardial infarction or ischemia, Digoxin toxicity, heart failure, cardiac surgery, valvular heart disease
Treatment	• Treatment of underlying cause • Drugs like Beta-blockers, Calcium channel blockers and Adenosine

Table 3.2 Junctional tachycardia

- This is a form of supraventricular tachycardia in which *enhanced automaticity of the AV node* generates fast impulses that essentially suppress the SA node.

AV Nodal Re-entry Tachycardia (AVNRT)

- Most common type of paroxysmal supraventricular tachycardia.
- This rhythm originates because of the presence of distinct slow and fast pathways within the AV node, possessing two distinct depolarization properties
- **Fast pathway** has *longer refractory time* and **slow pathway**

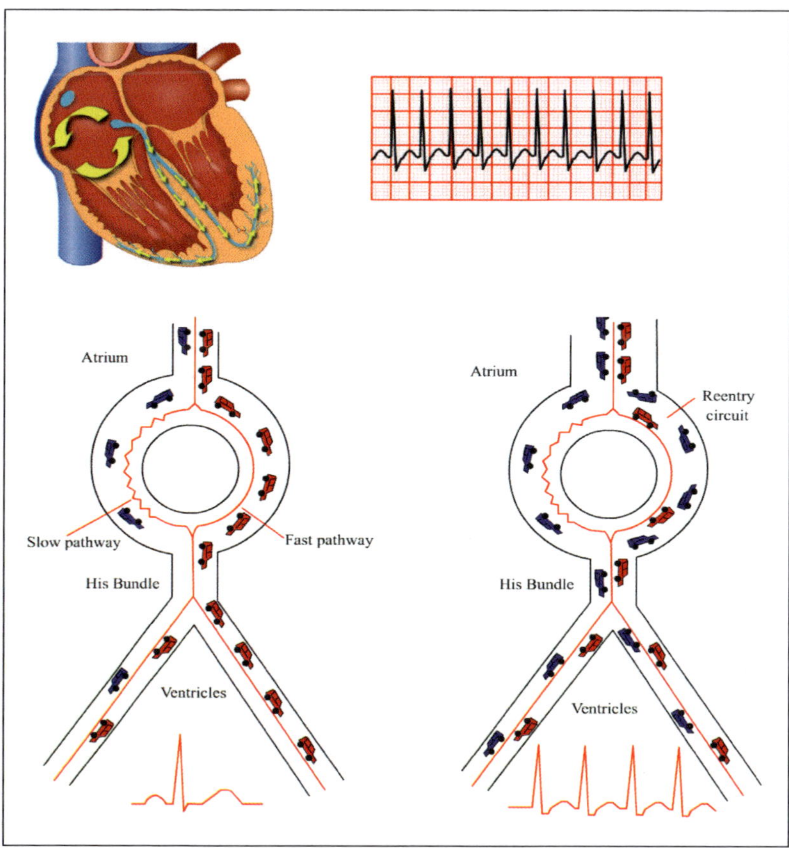

Fig 3.2 AVNRT mechanism

with *shorter refractory period.*

- During *normal sinus rhythm*, *only fast pathway* is manifested in an EKG even though impulses pass through both fast and slow pathways

- A premature atrial contraction (PAC) originating at a critical moment during cardiac cycle may be blocked in the fast pathway because of their longer refractory period. However, relatively shorter refractory period of the slow pathway may allow this impulse to conduct through slow pathway alone. During this slow conduction phase, the fast pathways comes out of their refractory period and therefore available for

AV Nodal Re-entry Tachycardia (AVNRT)

Rhythm	Regular
Rate	120-250 beats per minute
P wave	Inverted, absent or trailing
PR interval	Longer in the initiating impulse. Unable to measure if P wave is absent.
QRS complex	Narrow and regular
T wave	Regular or distorted by buried P wave.
QT interval	Normal or varying depending on the T wave.
Clinical significance	In the absence of structural heart disease, AVNRT usually is asymptomatic. In presence of coexisting structural heart disease, this rhythm may produce *hypotension* or *syncope*.
Causes	Common in females and may occur in absence of structural heart disease
Treatment	• Vagal maneuvers, Adenosine, Beta-blockers or Calcium channel blockers. • Synchronized DC cardioversion • Radiofrequency ablation of slow pathway

Table 3.3 AV nodal re-entry tachycardia

impulse conduction. The impulse that is conducting through the slow pathway may then get in to the fast pathway circuit and start retrograde conduction, leading to a vicious *re-entry pathway within the AV node*.

- The characteristic EKG finding in AVNRT is the *long PR interval of PAC initiating this rhythm*, suggesting *impulse conduction through slow pathway*

- Similar to any other junctional rhythm, P waves may either be inverted (retrograde conduction) or absent (buried in T wave).

Wolff- Parkinson-White Syndrome (WPW)

- In WPW syndrome, there is existence of abnormal connection or an **accessory pathway** between the atria and the ventricle known as **Bundle of Kent**.

- WPW is also known as **pre-excitation syndrome**.

- This short circuit allows conducting *some impulses to the ventricle before AV node does it* or *allowing impulses to enter back to the atria from the ventricle*. This re-entry circuit can create **re-entry tachycardia**.

- The retrograde activation of the atria through accessory pathway is known as **echo beat**.

- Since this accessory pathway does not extend throughout the ventricle like the **His-Purkinje system**, impulse travelling through accessory pathway *cannot initiate a complete ventricular contraction.* So in the resulting EKG, a characteristic *slurring of initial portion of QRS* known as **Delta wave** will be present in some patients.

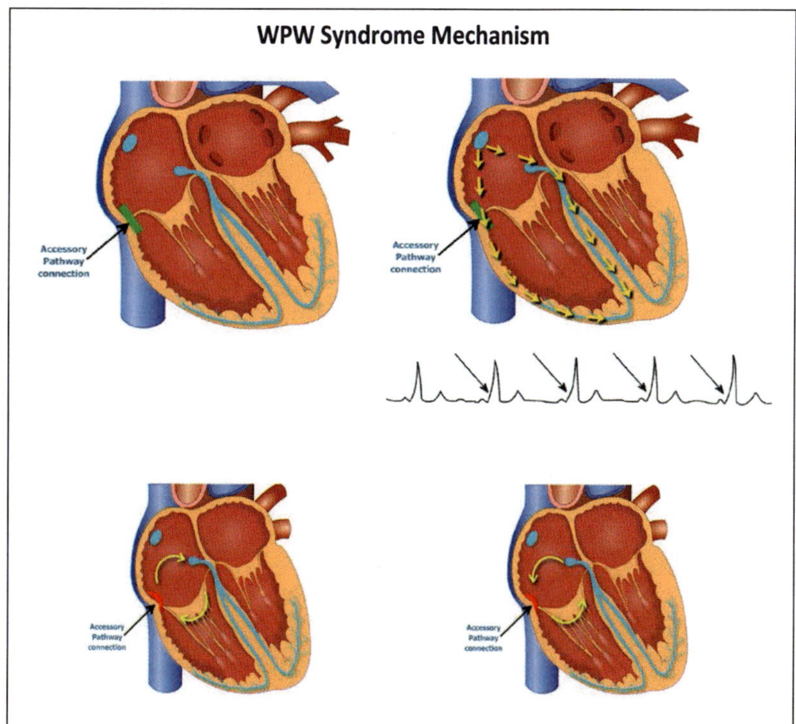

Fig 3.3 WPW syndrome mechanism

- Some impulses bypass the AV node through this fast pathway and result in a short PR interval.
- *Atrial fibrillation with WPW can create a wide QRS complex tachycardia* resembling V-tach
- The major differentiation between ventricular tachycardia and atrial fibrillation with WPW is that *ventricular tachycardia is usually regular* and *atrial fib with WPW is irregular*.
- WPW syndrome is associated with congenital anomalies such as **Ebstein anomaly**, **mitral valve prolapse** and **hypertrophic cardiomyopathy** (**HCM**).
- These patients generally have AV nodal re-entry tachycardia (AVRT), atrial fibrillation or flutter.
- Asymptomatic patients with WPW do not need any treatment.
- Definite management of WPW is a **radiofrequency catheter ablation** of the re-entry pathway and is the primary treatment of choice
- Depending on the type of AVRT, *intravenous Beta-blockers* or *Procanamide* can be useful for suppression of tachycardia in acute phase.
- **Procanamide** is of special importance because of its ability to depress conduction and prolong refractoriness except that of the AV node.
- For patients with infrequent episodes of AVRT, *Propafenone* and *Flecainide* can be used in long-term.

Atrioventricular block

- In normal conduction system of the heart, impulses originating from the SA node spread across the atria and channels down to

Heart Block

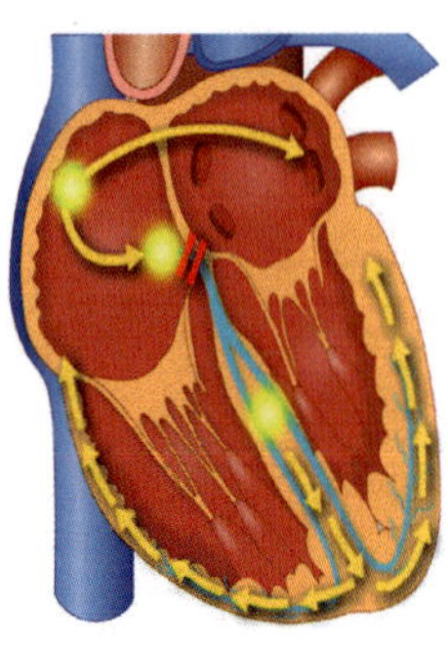

Fig 3.4 Various types of heart block

the AV node.

- At the AV node, these impulses are delayed due to so-called **decremental conduction** and thereby allowing atrial depolarization.

- During atrioventricular block, this *delaying mechanism becomes so profound* that either the *delay at the AV junction increases* or some of the atrial beats *do not conduct* down to the ventricle.

First-Degree Heart Block

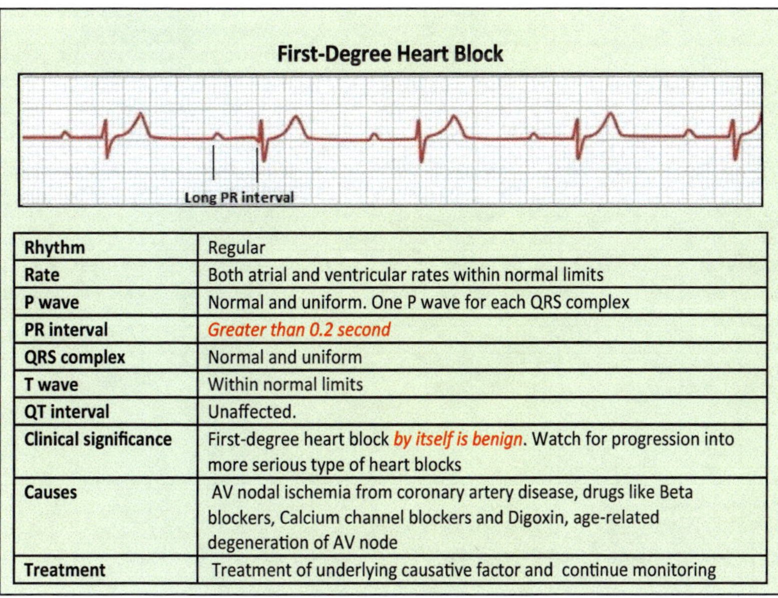

First-Degree Heart Block

Long PR interval

Rhythm	Regular
Rate	Both atrial and ventricular rates within normal limits
P wave	Normal and uniform. One P wave for each QRS complex
PR interval	*Greater than 0.2 second*
QRS complex	Normal and uniform
T wave	Within normal limits
QT interval	Unaffected.
Clinical significance	First-degree heart block *by itself is benign*. Watch for progression into more serious type of heart blocks
Causes	AV nodal ischemia from coronary artery disease, drugs like Beta blockers, Calcium channel blockers and Digoxin, age-related degeneration of AV node
Treatment	Treatment of underlying causative factor and continue monitoring

Table 3.4 First-degree heart block

- More than usual delay in conduction through the AV node creates the hallmark EKG change in first-degree heart block as *elongated PR interval*.

- Even though an increased delay exists, *all the impulses get through AV node* and complete their conduction.

Second-Degree Type I Heart Block (Wenckebach)

- There is a *periodic conduction failure* within the AV node causing *PR interval to progressively lengthen until a drop in QRS complex*.

- Unlike first-degree heart block, *all the atrial beats do not conduct to ventricle during* **Wenckebach phenomena**

Second-Degree Type II Heart Block (Mobitz Type II)

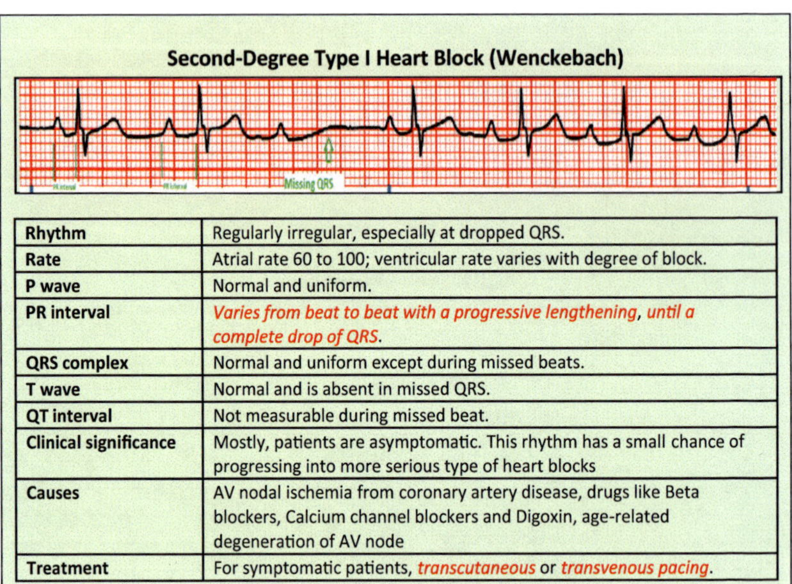

Second-Degree Type I Heart Block (Wenckebach)

Rhythm	Regularly irregular, especially at dropped QRS.
Rate	Atrial rate 60 to 100; ventricular rate varies with degree of block.
P wave	Normal and uniform.
PR interval	*Varies from beat to beat with a progressive lengthening*, *until a complete drop of QRS*.
QRS complex	Normal and uniform except during missed beats.
T wave	Normal and is absent in missed QRS.
QT interval	Not measurable during missed beat.
Clinical significance	Mostly, patients are asymptomatic. This rhythm has a small chance of progressing into more serious type of heart blocks
Causes	AV nodal ischemia from coronary artery disease, drugs like Beta blockers, Calcium channel blockers and Digoxin, age-related degeneration of AV node
Treatment	For symptomatic patients, *transcutaneous* or *transvenous pacing*.

Table 3.5 Second-degree type I heart block

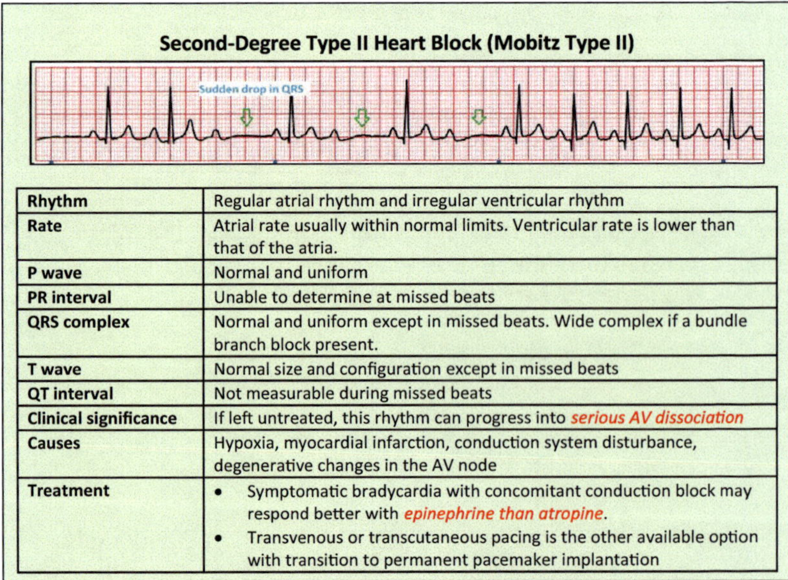

Second-Degree Type II Heart Block (Mobitz Type II)

Rhythm	Regular atrial rhythm and irregular ventricular rhythm
Rate	Atrial rate usually within normal limits. Ventricular rate is lower than that of the atria.
P wave	Normal and uniform
PR interval	Unable to determine at missed beats
QRS complex	Normal and uniform except in missed beats. Wide complex if a bundle branch block present.
T wave	Normal size and configuration except in missed beats
QT interval	Not measurable during missed beats
Clinical significance	If left untreated, this rhythm can progress into *serious AV dissociation*
Causes	Hypoxia, myocardial infarction, conduction system disturbance, degenerative changes in the AV node
Treatment	• Symptomatic bradycardia with concomitant conduction block may respond better with *epinephrine than atropine*. • Transvenous or transcutaneous pacing is the other available option with transition to permanent pacemaker implantation

Table 3.6 Second-degree type II heart block

- Characteristic EKG shows *a regular rhythm with constant PR interval from beat to beat until a* **sudden drop of complete QRS complex**.
- There is a high likeliness that this *rhythm can progress to the third-degree heart block*
- Occasionally, the block can be seen in regular pattern such as 2:1 or 3:1 conduction

Third Degree AV Block (AV Dissociation)

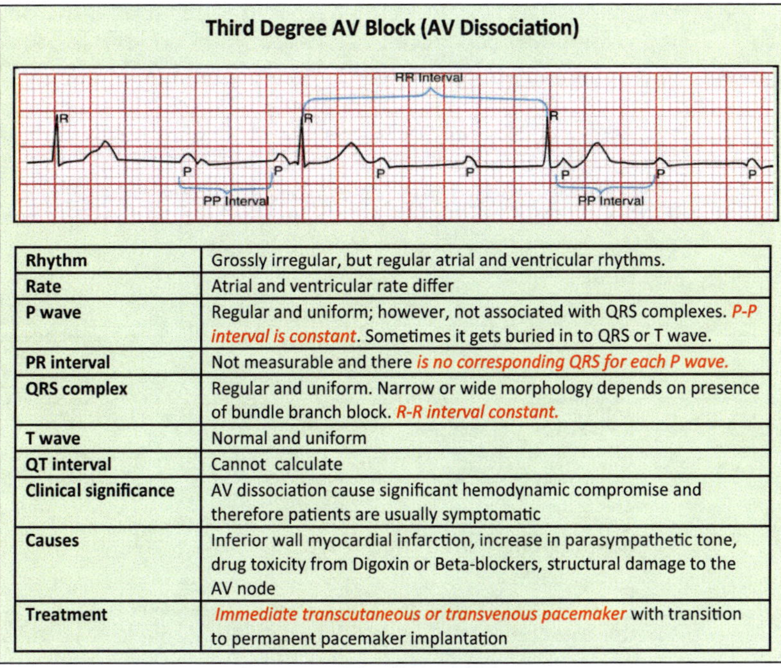

Third Degree AV Block (AV Dissociation)

Rhythm	Grossly irregular, but regular atrial and ventricular rhythms.
Rate	Atrial and ventricular rate differ
P wave	Regular and uniform; however, not associated with QRS complexes. *P-P interval is constant*. Sometimes it gets buried in to QRS or T wave.
PR interval	Not measurable and there *is no corresponding QRS for each P wave.*
QRS complex	Regular and uniform. Narrow or wide morphology depends on presence of bundle branch block. *R-R interval constant.*
T wave	Normal and uniform
QT interval	Cannot calculate
Clinical significance	AV dissociation cause significant hemodynamic compromise and therefore patients are usually symptomatic
Causes	Inferior wall myocardial infarction, increase in parasympathetic tone, drug toxicity from Digoxin or Beta-blockers, structural damage to the AV node
Treatment	*Immediate transcutaneous or transvenous pacemaker* with transition to permanent pacemaker implantation

Table 3.7 Third degree AV block

- During third-degree heart block, there is no electrical connection between upper and lower chambers and therefore **no synchronized contraction**.
- Here, atria *contracts at one rate* and *ventricles contract at a different rate*.
- Since there is no synchronization between these chamber contractions, serious hemodynamic compromise can occur immediately.

4 Ventricular Rhythms

- Ventricular rhythms are originated from an ectopic focus within the ventricle and generate *wide and bizarre QRS complexes* with duration **more than 0.12 seconds**.
- Most of these impulses don't have an atrial component and some of them have retrograde conduction to atria.
- Some of this retrograde conduction from ventricular beats combined with antegrade SA node conduction creates **fusion beats**.
- Fusion beats can be distinguished from other PVCs because, *it happens at the exact timing as a normal SA nodal beat* supposed to occur and has *different shape* compared to other PVCs
- Because of the disorganized ventricular depolarization, the *T wave usually assumes opposite direction of the QRS complex* during ventricular rhythms
- Because of the lack of effective atrial contraction and disorganized ventricular depolarization, these rhythms may not provide adequate cardiac output
- Ventricular pacemaker cells have an inherent pacing rate of **20 to 40 bpm**

Premature Ventricular Contraction (PVC)

- Premature ventricular contractions are ectopic beats originate within the ventricle and are mostly benign in nature.
- If they originate from a single focus, they are uniform in appearance (**unifocal**). Waves with varying morphology (Multifocal) are seen in rhythms originating from multiple

foci.

- Sometimes they occur at regular intervals such as every other

Differentiation Between PAC with Aberrancy and PVC

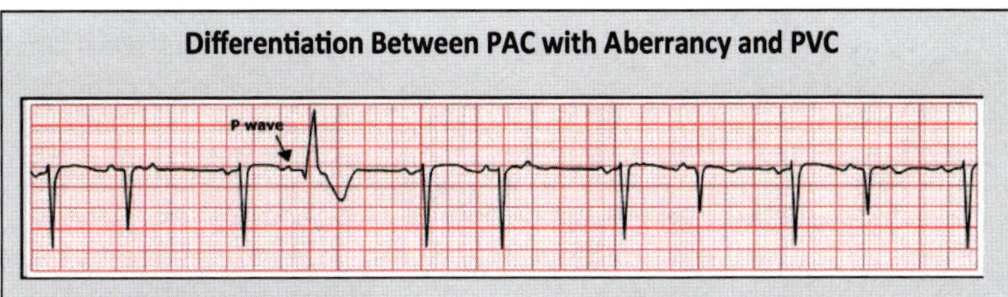

Premature atrial contraction with aberrant conduction may also produce wide and bizarre QRS complex that needs to be distinguished from that of ventricular tachycardia. *Presence of a premature P wave at the beginning of tachyarrhythmia* or *typical right or left bundle branch block pattern of QRS complex* are the tell-tale signs of differentiating **PAC with aberrant conduction** from that of **Ventricular tachycardia** (**V-tach**). Note the presence of p wave before distorted QRS complex in the picture.

Box 4.1 Differentiation between PAC with aberrancy and PVC

beat (**bigeminy**), every third beat (**trigeminy** or in pairs known as **couplets**.

Premature Ventricular Contraction (PVC)

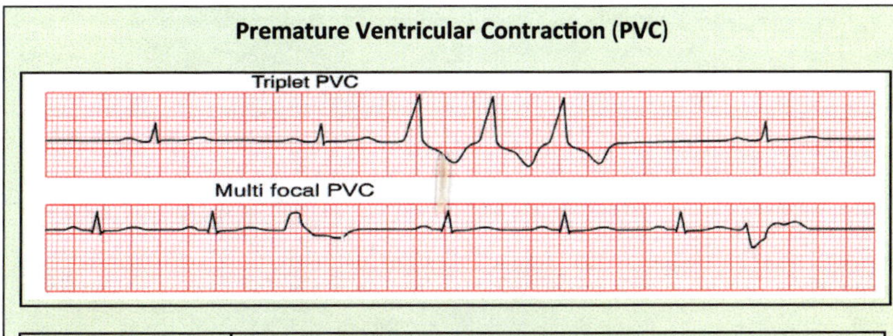

Rhythm	Underlying regular rhythm with irregularity during PVC.
Rate	Usually within normal limits.
P wave	Normal except during PVC, where it is absent.
PR interval	Normal except during PVC, where it is immeasurable.
QRS complex	*Wide and bizarre*, with *duration >0.12 second* during PVC
T wave	*Points to the opposite direction of QRS deflection* (if QRS negative, T wave positive).
QT interval	Not measurable during PVC
Clinical significance	Occasional PVCs are benign. If they occur more frequently, especially in the setting of underlying structural heart disease, it can progress to lethal ventricular tachycardia or fibrillation
Causes	Advanced age, structural heart disease, electrolyte imbalance, acidosis, congestive heart failure, acute myocardial infarction, drug toxicity
Treatment	• Management of underlying disease process • Drugs like Amiodarone, Lidocaine, Beta-blockers and Procanamide. • If the rhythm progress into ventricular tachycardia, electrical defibrillation and establishment of ICD for long-term prevention of sudden cardiac death (SCD)

Table 4.1 Premature ventricular contraction

- If there are *more than three beats in a row*, it is termed as a **run of VT**.

- Mostly there is complete or incomplete compensatory pause following PVCs since the retrograde conduction of the ventricular impulse can cancel out the atrial stimuli coming down through the AV node.

Idioventricular Rhythm

- This is a true ventricular rhythm with a rate of **20 to 40 bpm** and is a telltale sign of *imminent life-threatening events* like

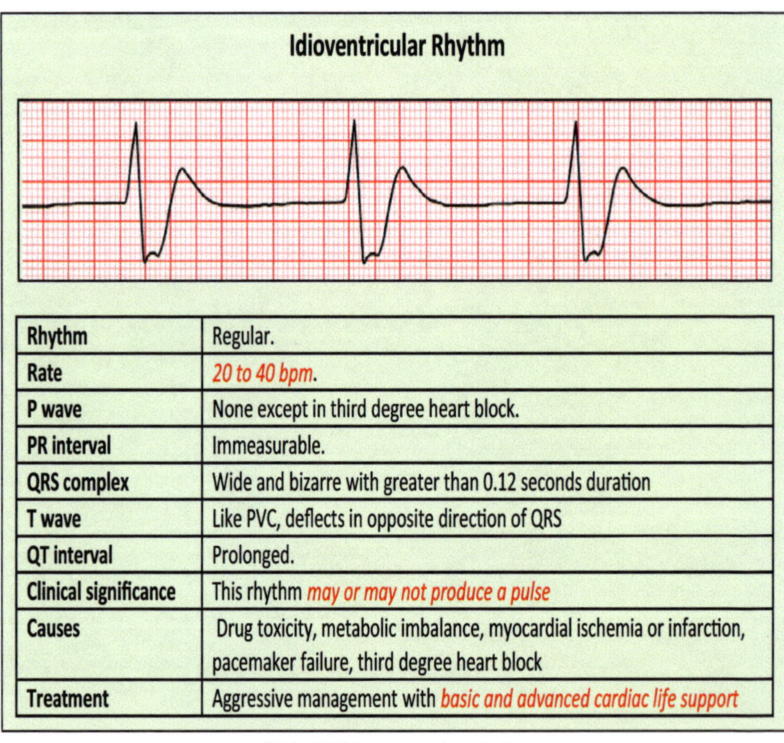

Idioventricular Rhythm

Rhythm	Regular.
Rate	*20 to 40 bpm*.
P wave	None except in third degree heart block.
PR interval	Immeasurable.
QRS complex	Wide and bizarre with greater than 0.12 seconds duration
T wave	Like PVC, deflects in opposite direction of QRS
QT interval	Prolonged.
Clinical significance	This rhythm *may or may not produce a pulse*
Causes	Drug toxicity, metabolic imbalance, myocardial ischemia or infarction, pacemaker failure, third degree heart block
Treatment	Aggressive management with *basic and advanced cardiac life support*

Table 4.2 Idioventricular rhythm

agonal rhythm or *asystole*.

- This is also known as **ventricular escape rhythm** and usually happens when all the higher-level pacemakers have failed.

- At times, this rhythm accompanies *complete AV dissociation* (third degree heart block).

Agonal Rhythm

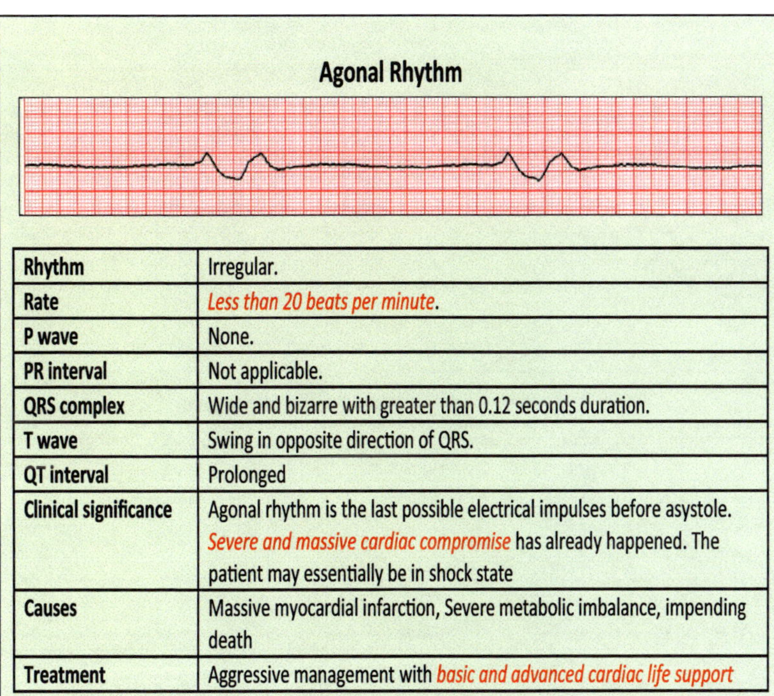

Agonal Rhythm

Rhythm	Irregular.
Rate	*Less than 20 beats per minute*.
P wave	None.
PR interval	Not applicable.
QRS complex	Wide and bizarre with greater than 0.12 seconds duration.
T wave	Swing in opposite direction of QRS.
QT interval	Prolonged
Clinical significance	Agonal rhythm is the last possible electrical impulses before asystole. *Severe and massive cardiac compromise* has already happened. The patient may essentially be in shock state
Causes	Massive myocardial infarction, Severe metabolic imbalance, impending death
Treatment	Aggressive management with *basic and advanced cardiac life support*

Table 4.3 Agonal rhythm

- This is the *worst possible cardiac rhythm second to asystole*. It denotes severely impaired cardiac function with impending death.

- Characterized by irregular occasional wide complex beats.

Accelerated Idioventricular Rhythm (AIVR)

- Accelerated Idioventricular rhythm originates due to *abnormal automaticity* within the ventricle and produce impulse at **40 to 120 bpm**.

- The basic characteristic that differentiates **AIVR** from that of **slow V-tach** is its *gradual onset and termination with a brief self-limiting pattern*.

- In order to differentiate **Idioventricular rhythm** (**IVR**) from A**ccelerated Idioventricular rhythm** (**AIVR**), *look for presence of P waves in AIVR that is absent in Idioventricular escape rhythm*.

Accelerated Idioventricular Rhythm (AIVR)

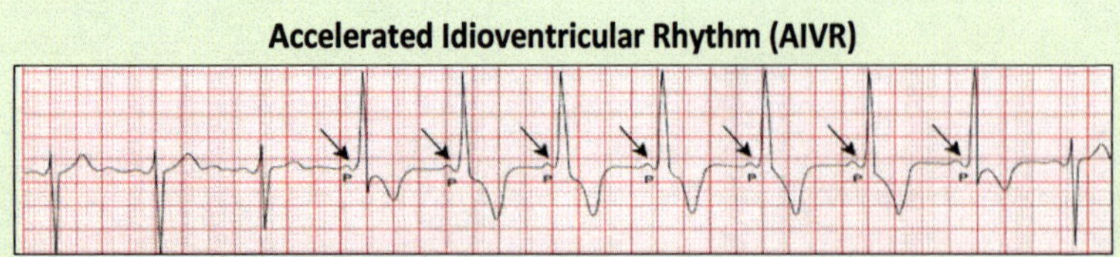

Rhythm	Mostly regular
Rate	*40 to 120 bpm.*
P wave	May be seen *before, during* or *after QRS*. At times, *inverted* or *absent*
PR interval	Immeasurable if P waves are absent
QRS complex	*Wide and bizarre*, duration >.12 seconds
T wave	Wide
QT interval	Prolonged
Clinical significance	Hemodynamic compromise rarely occurs with AIVR. Mostly it is a self-limiting arrhythmia.
Causes	It can be seen in the absence of any structural heart disease or in the event of acute myocardial infarction, cocaine toxicity, Digoxin intoxication, postoperative cardiac surgery or after *chemical or mechanical revascularization of coronary arteries* as in **tPA administration** and **coronary angioplasty**. In these settings, it is also known as **reperfusion arrhythmia**.
Treatment	If asymptomatic, no treatment is needed. Correct underlying causative factors.

Table 4.4 Accelerated idioventricular rhythm

- In **AIVR,** *SA node is still firing* unlike in **IVR** where there is no functioning higher order pacemaker.

- Because of the rate at which the ventricles contract, mostly *AIVR does not produce significant compromise in cardiac output*.

Ventricular Tachycardia

- There are *three or more PVCs in a row* and *ventricular rate exceeds 100 bpm*.

- If the duration of ventricular tachycardia is less than 30 seconds, it is called **non-sustained ventricular tachycardia (NSVT).**

- If the rhythm *persists for more than 30 seconds* or terminated within 30 seconds by either An Implantable Defibrillator (**ICD** or **AICD**) or external defibrillation, it is known as **sustained VT**.

- Depending on the morphologic characteristics, VT can be classified into **monomorphic VT** and **polymorphic VT**.

Ventricular Tachycardia

Rhythm	Usually regular.
Rate	*Ventricular rate between 100 to 250 bpm*; atrial rhythm is indiscernible.
P wave	Usually absent or indistinguishable
PR interval	Not applicable.
QRS complex	*Wide and bizarre* with the duration >0.12 seconds.
T wave	In the opposite direction of QRS deflection.
QT interval	Prolonged.
Clinical significance	Depending on the duration and frequency of ventricular tachycardia, it may be well tolerable or having serious hemodynamic effects. Since the contraction of ventricles at 150 to 250 bpm *does not provide time for effective ventricular contraction*; *cardiac output is considerably reduced*.
Causes	Cardiomyopathy, electrolyte imbalance, heart failure, myocardial ischemia and infarction, valvular heart disease, drug toxicity, re-entry arrhythmia.
Treatment	• VT or V-Fib that is compromising hemodynamic function should be treated with immediate **asynchronous DC cardioversion**. • Intravenous **Lidocaine** or **Amiodarone**. • ICD implantation for prevention of sudden cardiac death.

Table 4.5 Ventricular tachycardia

- Repeated ventricular tachycardia episodes requiring electrical cardioversion or defibrillation with *more than two incidents within 24 hours* are defined as **VT storm**.

Torsades de Pointes (TDP)

- A form of **polymorphic ventricular tachycardia** with a *varying QRS morphology*. It has an *undulating QRS complex* with reference to the isoelectric line.
- This can degenerate into **ventricular fibrillation** with serious hemodynamic compromise.
- TDP refers to a more serious unstable situation, urgent treatment is warranted.

Ventricular Fibrillation (V Fib)

- A *completely disorganized and chaotic ventricular rhythm* that has serious hemodynamic implications.
- Multiple ectopic foci within the ventricle start firing impulses; leading to unsystematic depolarization of the ventricles.
- Resultant 'quivering' motion of ventricles essentially produce

Torsades de Pointes (TDP)

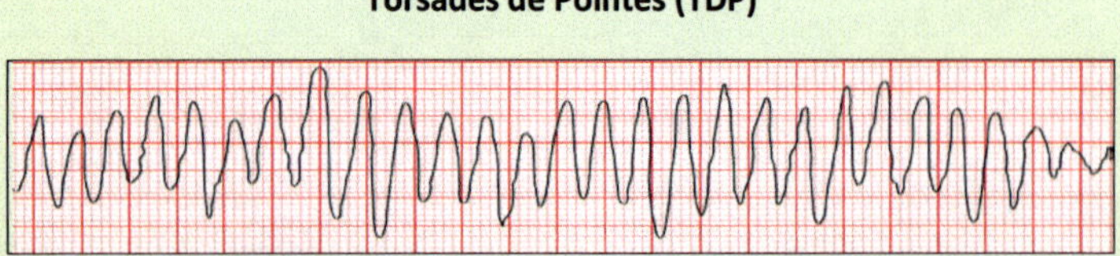

Rhythm	May be regular or irregular with varying QRS size.
Rate	Atrial rate immeasurable, ventricular rate 150 to 300 bpm.
P wave	Not seen.
PR interval	Unable to calculate.
QRS complex	Wide and bizarre with the duration greater than 0.12 seconds. Complexes with positive and negative deflection are present compared to isoelectric line.
T wave	Difficult to identify.
QT interval	Prolonged in beats prior to torsades.
Clinical significance	Considered as one of the lethal arrhythmias since it can degrade into ventricular fibrillation. *Short runs of torsades are generally well tolerated* in the absence of critical hemodynamic issues.
Causes	Acute ischemia, myocarditis, hypomagnesaemia, pro arrhythmic drugs like Procainamide and Amiodarone.
Treatment	• Intravenous magnesium. • Asynchronous DC cardioversion. • Intravenous Lidocaine or Amiodarone

Table 4.6 Torsades de Pointes

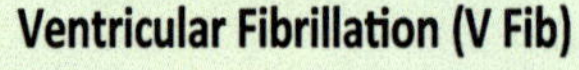

Ventricular Fibrillation (V Fib)

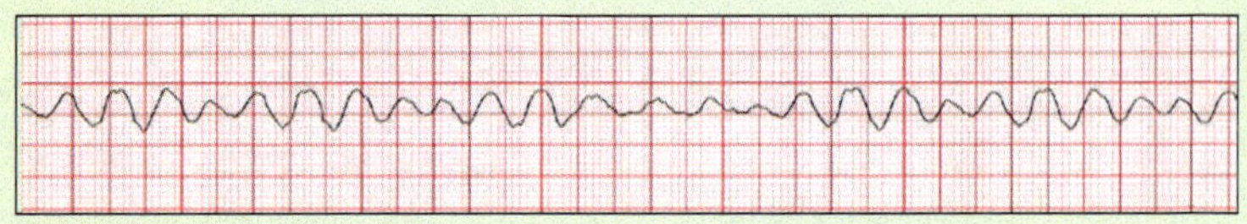

Rhythm	*Completely irregular*, *with fibrillatory waves*.
Rate	Cannot be determined.
P wave	Not seen.
PR interval	Cannot calculate.
QRS complex	No definite QRS; *just undulating waves*.
T wave	Not seen.
QT interval	Cannot calculate
Clinical significance	This rhythm does not generate any cardiac output whatsoever.
Causes	Metabolic imbalance, myocardial ischemia or infarction, severe hypothermia, cardiomyopathy, untreated ventricular tachycardia
Treatment	• Immediate basic and advanced life support measures including defibrillation. • **Amiodarone** and **Lidocaine** are used after electrical defibrillation to prevent recurrence of VT/V fib.

Table 4.7 Ventricular fibrillation

ventricular standstill.

- V fib can be with coarse or *fine fibrillatory waves*.

Asystole

- This denotes a *complete ventricular standstill* with no cardiac output.
- In the EKG, a **flat line** appears and it essentially means there is absolutely no pacemaker activity happening anywhere in the heart.

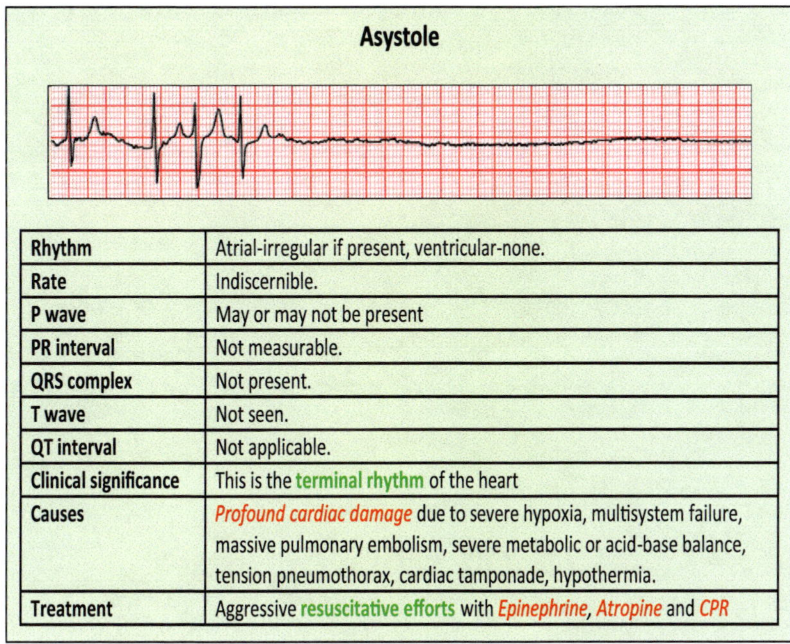

Asystole

Rhythm	Atrial-irregular if present, ventricular-none.
Rate	Indiscernible.
P wave	May or may not be present
PR interval	Not measurable.
QRS complex	Not present.
T wave	Not seen.
QT interval	Not applicable.
Clinical significance	This is the **terminal rhythm** of the heart
Causes	*Profound cardiac damage* due to severe hypoxia, multisystem failure, massive pulmonary embolism, severe metabolic or acid-base balance, tension pneumothorax, cardiac tamponade, hypothermia.
Treatment	Aggressive **resuscitative efforts** with *Epinephrine*, *Atropine* and *CPR*

Table 4.8 Asystole

- If the patient has a pacemaker either permanent or temporary, we may see pacing spikes at regular intervals without corresponding P or QRS complex.
-

5 Pacemakers and ICD

- Pacemakers are indicated for patients with various disorders of automaticity and conductivity.
- Based on the function, pacemakers can be divided into **Fixed** pacemakers and **Demand** pacemakers.
- **Fixed pacemakers** fires impulses to the designated chamber at a *fixed rate irrespective of the patient's innate cardiac activity*.
- **Demand pacemakers** are devices that generate impulses *based on the person's innate cardiac impulse*.
- These types of devices have a preset range of programming and the device *will pace only when the person's heart rate drops below the set rate*.
- Another classification is based on the number of chambers being paced. It can be **single chamber or a dual chamber** pacemaker.
- **Single chamber** pacemaker does *either sensing or pacing the atrium or the ventricle*.

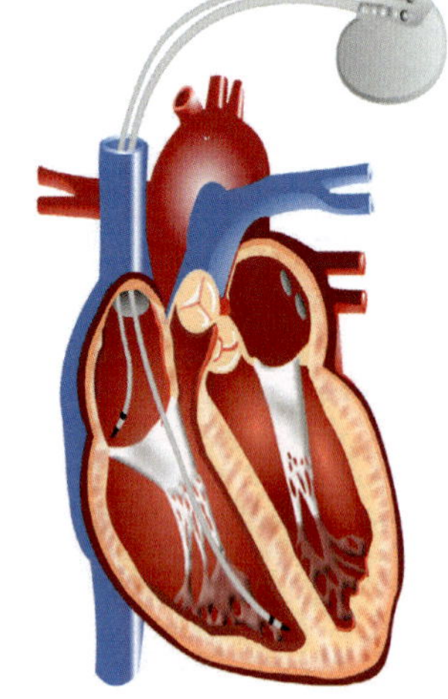

Fig 5.1 Dual chamber pacemaker

- **Dual chamber** with *pacing and sensing function in the atria and the ventricle* (both chambers).
- In patients with SA node dysfunction where there is deficiency in impulse production, an **atrial pacemaker** is helpful by providing much-needed electrical stimuli in the atria.
- In patients with conduction defect such as *complete heart block*, a *single chamber pacemaker does not work* because of the *lack of atrio-ventricular connection*.
- Here, the dual chamber pacemaker is used to provide **atrio-ventricular synchronization**.

Indications for Pacemakers

- Sinus bradycardia (rate less than 40 bpm with pauses)
- Complete atrio-ventricular block (third degree heart block)
- Symptomatic second-degree AV block
- Exercise induced second-degree or third-degree block
- Significant vasovagal symptoms
- Second-degree Type II AV block with wide QRS
- Idioventricular rhythm

Box 5.1 Indications for pacemakers

- **Biventricular pacemakers** are particularly useful in patients with *depressed ventricular ejection fraction* with *coexisting bundle branch block*.
- In this situation, Instead of *contracting together*, both ventricles *depolarize in sequence* due to the delay in impulse conduction secondary to bundle branch block.
- **Cardiac Resynchronization Therapy** (CRT) using biventricular pacemakers ensure *simultaneous contraction of both ventricles*.
- **Biventricular ICD** (**BiV ICD**) has both *pacemaker function which is continuous and defibrillator function for possible ventricular tachyarrhythmia emergencies* and is useful for patients having *high propensity for ventricular arrhythmia*

with coexisting LV dysfunction and a bundle branch block.

- Since the pacemaker leads are not generally placed on the left ventricle; in a BiV ICD, left ventricular lead is placed in the **coronary sinus**
- Depending on the duration of use, pacemakers can be **permanent** pacemakers or **temporary** pacemakers.
- **Temporary pacemakers** are usually inserted through femoral or jugular veins and are intended for short-term use while the patients are being stabilized.
- Most common reasons for temporary pacemaker insertion are *fulminant inferior wall myocardial infarction*, *post cardiac surgery*, *third degree AV block* etc.
- There is more chance for complications like *infection*, *bleeding* and *lead displacement* with temporary pacemakers.
- Alternate access sites for temporary pacing are **transcutaneous** (with large pads attached to skin), **epicardial** (during and immediately post cardiac surgery) and **transthoracic** (by insertion of a needle into the right ventricle and threading pacemaker wire in to the heart) route.
- **Permanent pacemakers** are indicated for long-term use with extremely long battery life (*average 5-8 years*).
- Permanent pacemaker leads that are implanted commonly through **right or left subclavian vein** into the myocardium.
- These leads are connected to the pacemaker generator unit, which is usually implanted in the **infraclavicular fossa** (underneath the clavicle) on non dominant side of the patient (under left clavicle for right handed patient).
- These devices can be programmed externally with the use of specialized magnetic probes.

Modes of pacing

- Modern pacemakers can be programmed in such a way that they can provide most individualistic treatment protocol for the given patient depending on underlying disease process.
- The **rate response mechanism** provides a *range of atrial beats* (e.g. 60-100bpm) *under which the pacemaker will try to*

match one QRS complex for each P wave.

- Rate response mechanism is particularly useful in patients with atrial fibrillation.
- If the atrial rate falls below 60 or it goes above 100, the pacemaker will provide a **pre-determined rate** of ventricular impulses to maintain circulation.
- This mechanism is particularly useful in patients with

Modes of Pacing	
First letter	**Chamber Paced**
V	Ventricle
A	Atria
D	Dual or both
0	None
Second letter	**Chamber sensed**
V	Ventricle
A	Atria
D	Dual (Atria and Ventricle)
0	None
Third letter	**Pacemaker response to intrinsic rhythm**
T	Triggered (trigger pacing in response to a sensed event)
I	Inhibit (inhibits pacing in response to a sensed event)
D	Dual (It can inhibit and trigger impulses in various chambers depending on the event)
0	None(It does not respond to the sensed event)
Forth letter	**Rate response**
R	Rate responsive (pacemaker provide paced impulse for a pre-determined range of heart rate)
0	No rate response
Fifth letter	**Pacemaker's response to tachyarrhythmia**
P	Override pacing for tachycardia available
S	Shock therapy(available in high-energy devices e.g. AICD)
D	Dual-ability to pace and shock
0	None

Box 5.2 Modes of pacing

uncontrolled atrial rates; however, need to increase their heart rate during physical activity and exertion.

Complications of Pacemaker Therapy

- The EKG will show *pacer spikes at regular intervals* denoting normal functioning pacemaker with *no trailing P or QRS complexes* known as **failure to capture**. Here, the myocardium did not capture the impulse given by the pacemaker.

- Common causes for capture failure are *lead malfunction*, increased energy requirement for myocardial stimulation (*increased pacer threshold*) secondary to *metabolic* or

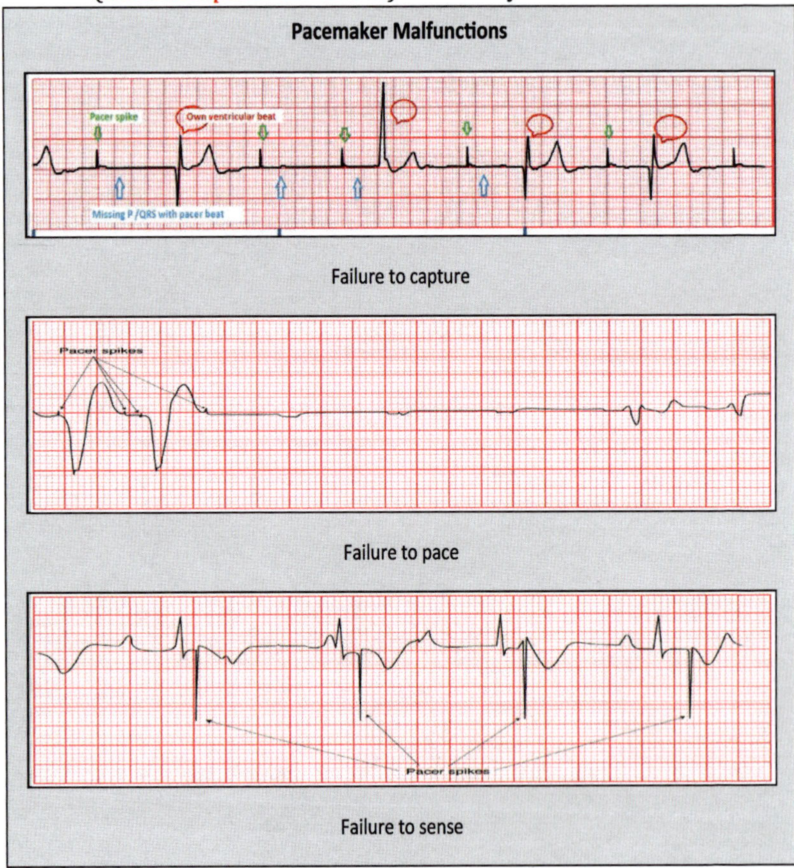

Box 5.3 Pacemaker malfunctions

electrolyte imbalance, *fibrosis of myocardium* at the site of lead insertion and use of *antiarrhythmic drugs* (increase pacer threshold).

- **Failure to Pace** is evident in the EKG as *missed beats when pacemaker was supposed to initiate an impulse*. If left untreated, this rhythm is dangerous as it essentially jeopardizes the reason for having a pacemaker in the first place.

- Probable causes for failure to pace include *weak battery*, *lead failure*, programming issues such as *poor sensing* and *electromagnetic interference (EMI)*.

- In **Failure to Sense**, the pacemaker *does not sense the intrinsic impulse for which it was supposed to inhibit pacing function*. In EKG, there are *multiple pacer spikes irrespective of the patient's own impulses*.

- This is mostly caused by *under sensing*, *lead malfunction*, *electromagnetic interference* etc.

- If any of these pacer beats happen to strike on the **downward slope of T wave**, where ventricles are most vulnerable for lethal arrhythmias; **ventricular tachycardia** may result.

- During **Over Sensing**, the pacemaker can *misinterpret* muscle movements and normal cardiac waveforms like T wave as innate electrical impulses and can act inappropriately.

- Misinterpreting T waves as QRS complex and interpreting entire rhythm as tachycardia when the heart rate is within normal limits is commonly seen in high-energy devices like ICD; leading to **inappropriate shock therapy** from these devices in these situations.

- Most common *unsafe devises* for patients with pacemakers are *high-energy electromagnetic devices such as MRI scan, electrical generators, welding equipments etc.* Day to day appliances such as *cordless phones, cell phones and microwave ovens* are largely safe to use with pacemakers as long as there is a considerable distance from the devise.

6 12 Lead EKG Interpretation

- Individual leads provide only a single view of the three-dimensional heart.
- In order to have a comprehensive view of the electrical activity of the heart, 6 horizontal and 6 vertical plane leads are used in 12 lead EKG.
- The leads are generally grouped together based on their representation of different walls of the heart.

Steps in 12 Lead EKG Interpretation

Steps in 12 lead EKG Interpretation

1. **R**hythm
2. **A**xis
3. **B**undle branch block
4. **E**nlargement of chamber
5. **I**schemia or infarction
6. **O**ther abnormalities

Box 6.1 Steps in 12 lead EKG interpretation

- **Determine the rhythm**: Just like assessing a single lead EKG, *look for the presence of* **P** wave, **QRS** complex, **T** wave and *their characteristics* and *morphology*. *Heart rate*, *various intervals* and *presence of any ectopic beats* should be noted.
- **Determine overall axis**: Electrical axis of the EKG simply shows the *direction of electricity flow* within the heart. Normally it is directed towards **left and inferior** aspect of the heart (towards left ventricle).
- **Presence of block**: Assess for **bundle branch block** or

hemiblock

- Check for **chamber enlargement** or thickness (Hypertrophy).
- Check for **ischemia** or **infarction.**
- Look for **other abnormalities** like hyperkalemia, A-V dissociation etc.

Electrical Axis of the Heart

- Electrical axis simply means *overall direction of the electrical flow within the heart*.
- The *left ventricle, being the major pumping chamber and having the greatest muscle thickness*; *much of this current is flowing towards left ventricle* and essentially **left word and downward** direction.
- This direction is also known as **left word and inferior** and is the **normal axis** of the EKG.
- Some of the basic concepts of EKG are
- 1. Electricity flows ***towards positive electrode*** generates a ***positive*** *(upright)* deflection in the resulting EKG.
- 2. Individual leads in an EKG provides **single linear view** of electrical activity of the heart.

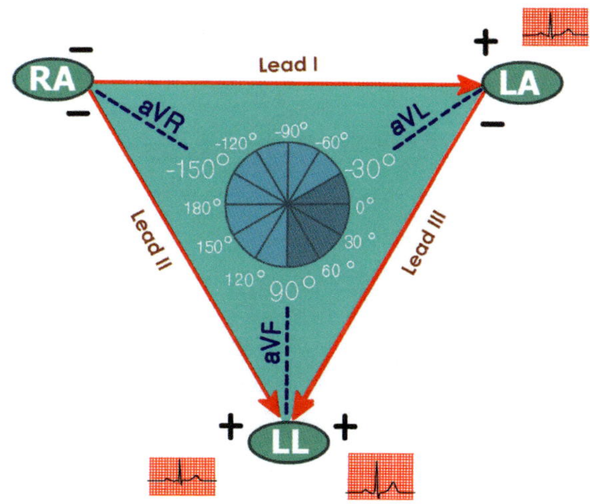

Fig 6.1 Frontal leads of EKG

- For Visualizing Axis in the Frontal Plane; lead **I**, **II**, **III**, **aVR**, **aVL** and **aVF** constitute the frontal plane leads in a 12 lead EKG.
- Lead **I** has a positive electrode on the left shoulder and negative electrode on the right. Therefore in lead **I,** an electrical activity travelling *towards left* will generate a *positive deflection* in the resulting EKG. Hence, lead **I** can be used in *differentiating impulses going towards **left*** (EKG with a positive wave) *from that going towards **right*** (a negative wave).

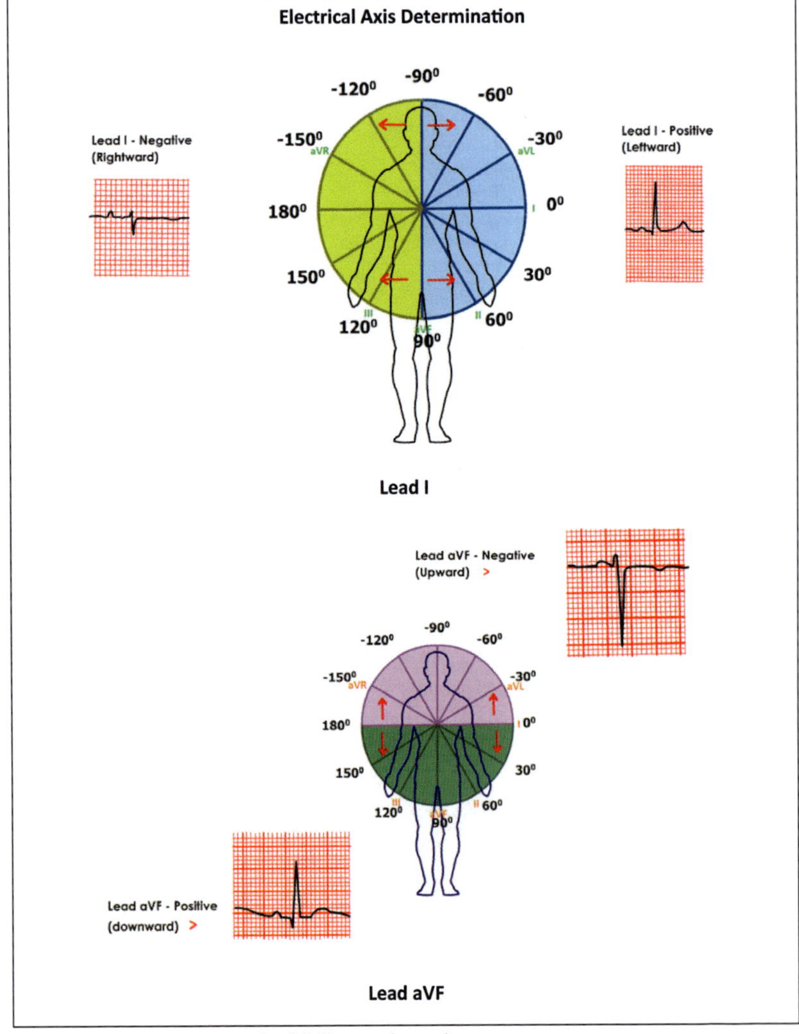

Fig 6.2 Electrical axis determination

- Similarly, lead **aVF** that is situated with a positive electrode on the left lower extremity; differentiate electricity going towards ***up*** or ***downward direction***.

- Even though a bit confusing, it is important to remember that when electricity flows **downward** (towards positive electrode), it produces a **positive waveform** in lead **aVF**.

- Conversely when **aVF** is **negative**, it denotes electricity

Simple Method for Right or Left Axis Determination

Lead	Normal Axis	Right axis deviation	Left axis deviation
I	Positive	Negative	Positive
II	Positive	Positive or Negative	Negative
III	Positive or Negative	Positive	Negative
aVF	Positive	Positive	Negative

Box 6.2 Simple method for right or left axis determination

flowing in **upward direction**.

- Once the vertical axis is determined, it is important to see the direction of electricity in the horizontal plane because of the three-dimensional structure of the heart.

- Normally the direction of flow of current is **towards the left ventricle** and that is towards **posterior** (remember, anatomically right ventricle is more towards the anterior chest wall).

- Flow of current in posterior direction is shown by a **positive wave** in lead **V6**, which is closer to the left ventricle (remember the position of **V6** electrode).

- Since lead **V1** and **V2** are situated in the anterior aspect of the chest wall, any flow of current in the anterior direction results in a positive waveform in these leads.

- The precordial leads are arranged in an *anterior to posterior* fashion so that they help to pinpoint the direction of electrical flow in the horizontal plane.

Coronary Circulation to the Conduction System

- In general, **right coronary artery** (**RCA**) supplies blood to the

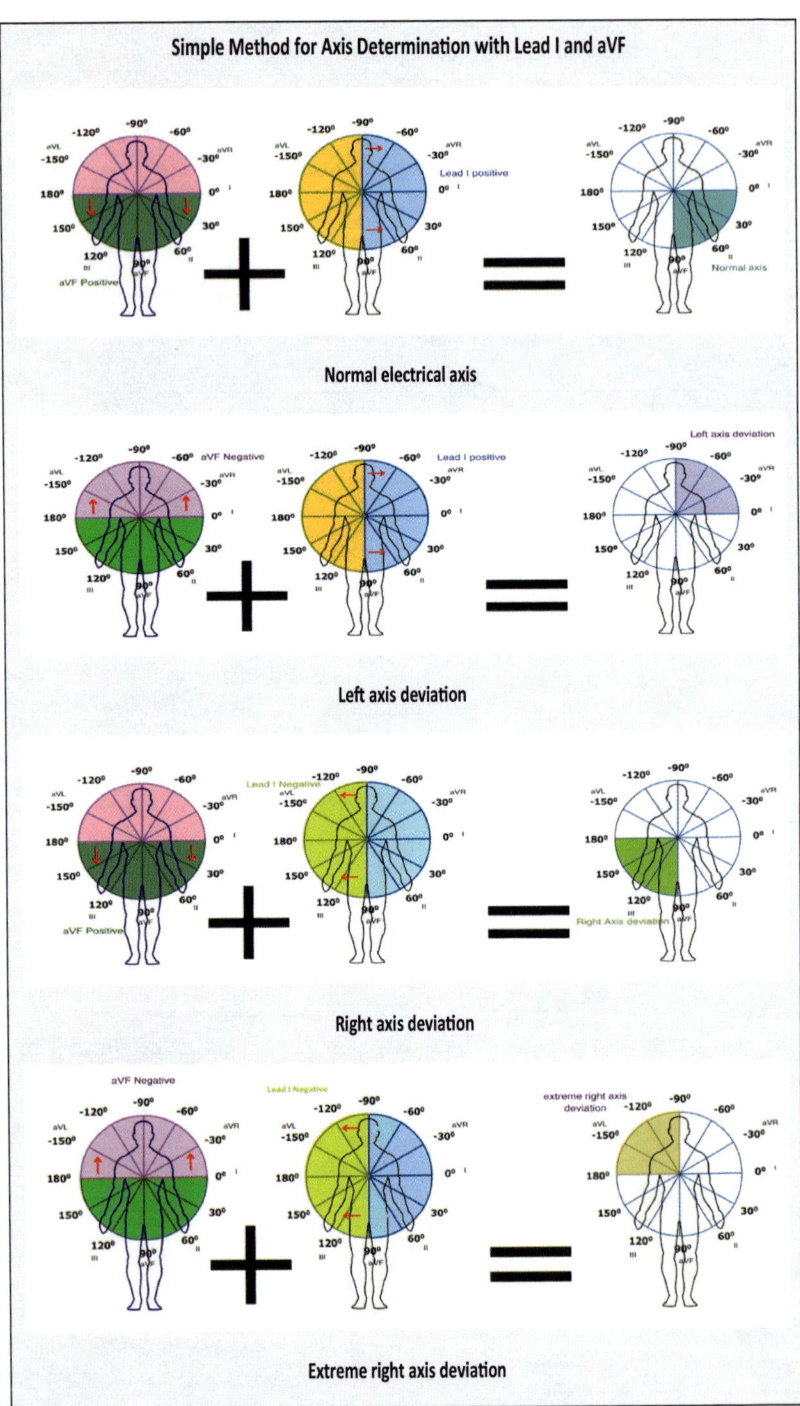

Fig 6.3 Method for axis determination with Lead I and aVF

proximal part of the conduction system including SA node and

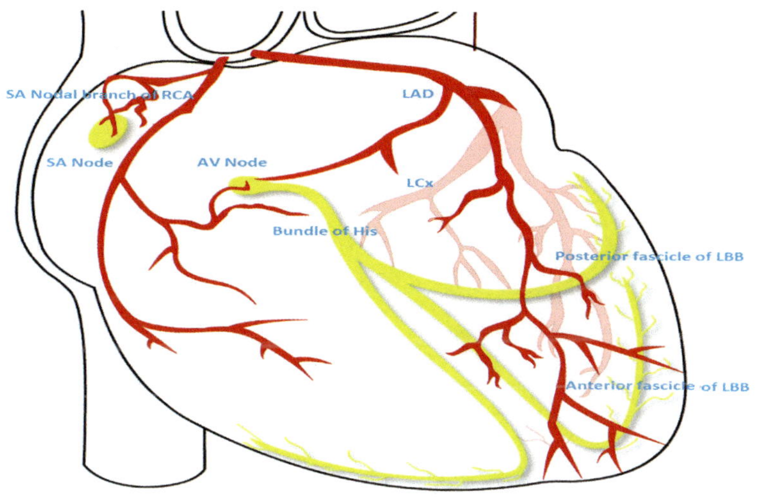

Fig 6.4 Coronary blood supply to the conduction system

AV node

- **Left anterior descending artery** (**LAD**) provides supply to *middle and distal aspects of the conduction system*.

- As a failsafe mechanism, some of the key elements of conduction system receive *dual blood supply* from two different arteries and that ensures adequate function of these areas in the event of the compromise of any one of the arteries.

- The **Sino atrial node** (**SA node**) is predominantly supplied by *branch of right coronary artery* called **SA nodal branch**.

- The *AV node and bundle of his* receive dual blood supply from both the *right coronary artery* (**RCA**) and *branch of left anterior descending artery* (**LAD**).

- *Left circumflex artery* provides blood supply to the *posterior fascicle of left bundle branch*.

- The distal aspect of the bundle branch as such as *right bundle branch and anterior fascicle of left bundle branch* receive blood supply from the *left anterior descending artery*.

Coronary Circulation to the Conduction System	
RCA	• SA node • AV node • Bundle of His • Posterior fascicle of Left bundle branch
LAD	• AV node • Bundle of His • Right bundle branch • Anterior fascicle of left bundle
LCx	• Posterior fascicle of Left bundle branch

Box 6.3 Coronary circulation to the conduction system

Right Bundle Branch Block

- The hallmark of any bundle branch block is *a wide QRS complex with duration greater than 0.12 seconds*. If the duration is between 0.10 seconds to the 0.11, it is called **Inter ventricular conduction delay** (**IVCD**).

- *Right ventricle is supplied by the right bundle branch* and *left ventricle by anterior and posterior fascicle of the left bundle* branch.

- When the right bundle is blocked, the only way right ventricle can get an impulse is from the left ventricle. However, this delay in conduction of impulse from left ventricle to the right ventricle causes the ventricles to contract *sequentially* (back to back) *rather than simultaneously* (together).

- In this situation, *rather than flowing towards the left ventricle that is leftward and posterior, the* **last part of QRS complex** *will be directing towards right ventricle*, *which is* ***anterior*** **and rightward**.

- Mainly lead **I**, **V1** and **V6** are considered in identifying **right bundle branch block** (**RBBB**).

- In right bundle branch block, the net direction of flow of current is towards right ventricle, which is *anterior and rightward*. Therefore, along with a wide QRS complex of duration greater than 0.12 seconds, *lead **I**, **V6** will be **negative*** and ***lead V1*** *will be* ***positive***.

- In general, **T waves are in opposite direction of QRS complex** because of the characteristic electricity flow of bundle branch block.

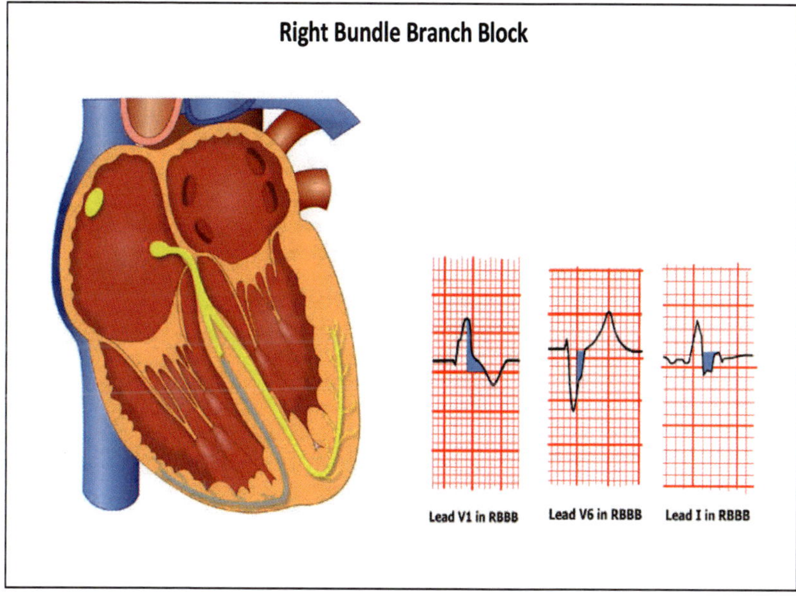

Fig 6.5 Right bundle branch block

- In an EKG with the right bundle branch block, *it is important to evaluate* **overall axis**, **ST segment elevation**, **myocardial infarction** and presence of **hemiblock**.

- Since the contraction of right bundle is sequential, this EKG is *not reliable for identifying right ventricle hypertrophy*.

Left Hemiblock

- Left bundle has two distinct bundle segments called left **anterior** or **superior fascicle** and left **posterior fascicle**.

- During *left anterior hemiblock*, *left anterior fascicle is blocked*. Left anterior hemiblock is also known as **left anterior superior hemiblock** (**LAHB**).

- In order to depolarize areas of myocardium covered by the anterior fascicle, the impulses spreading through posterior fascicle travel upward (towards anterior). This changes the axis of EKG in the frontal plane as evidenced by a **negative** aVF (remember, negative aVF means upward direction of current since aVF has positive electrode towards left leg). The mean direction of QRS in **LAHB** is therefore **leftward and upward**.

- Since part of the left bundle is still functioning, there *will not*

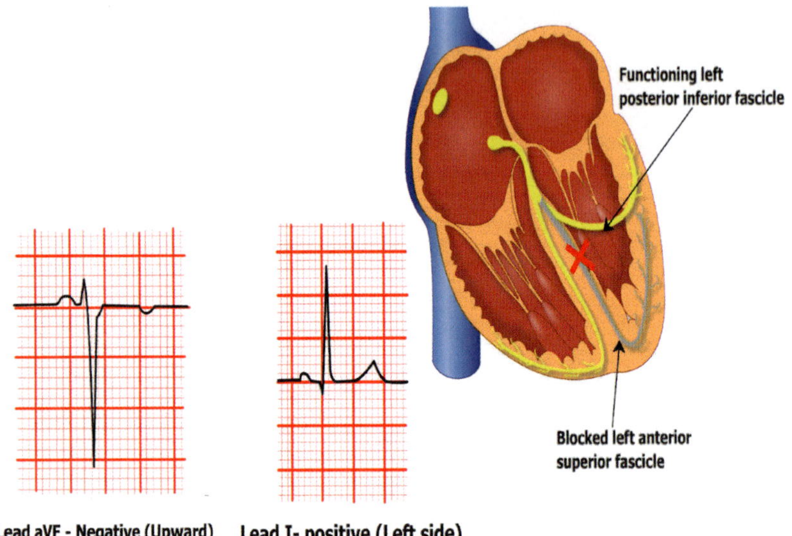

Fig 6.6 Left anterior or superior hemiblock

be any widening of QRS complex.

- However, this EKG may have a slight slurring of the QRS complex called **delayed intrinsicoid deflection** where the *time taken for the R wave to peak from the beginning of the QRS will be longer* than usual (>0.45 Sec or greater than 1 small box).

- Left anterior hemiblock has left axis deviation since ***aVL** is positive* and *lead **II**, **III*** and ***aVF** are negative*.

- In **left inferior** or **posterior hemiblock**, the direction of current will be from the anterior fascicle to the posterior fascicle and essentially **rightward and inferior**.

- So *lead **I** and **aVL** are negative* (rightward), *lead **II, III** and **aVF** are positive* (Inferior or downward). *Lead aVR is mostly isoelectric*, showing its perpendicular direction with the axis of EKG.

Left Bundle Branch Block

- In **left bundle branch block**, *the main left bundle before it's bifurcation in to anterior and posterior fascicle is blocked*.
- Here, the right ventricle contracts first from the electrical impulse through intact right bundle. Then the same impulse travels to the left ventricular myocardium, causing it to contract. Therefore during left bundle branch block, the right and left ventricles contract *sequentially rather than in tandem*.
- The direction of current is from *the right ventricle to the left*

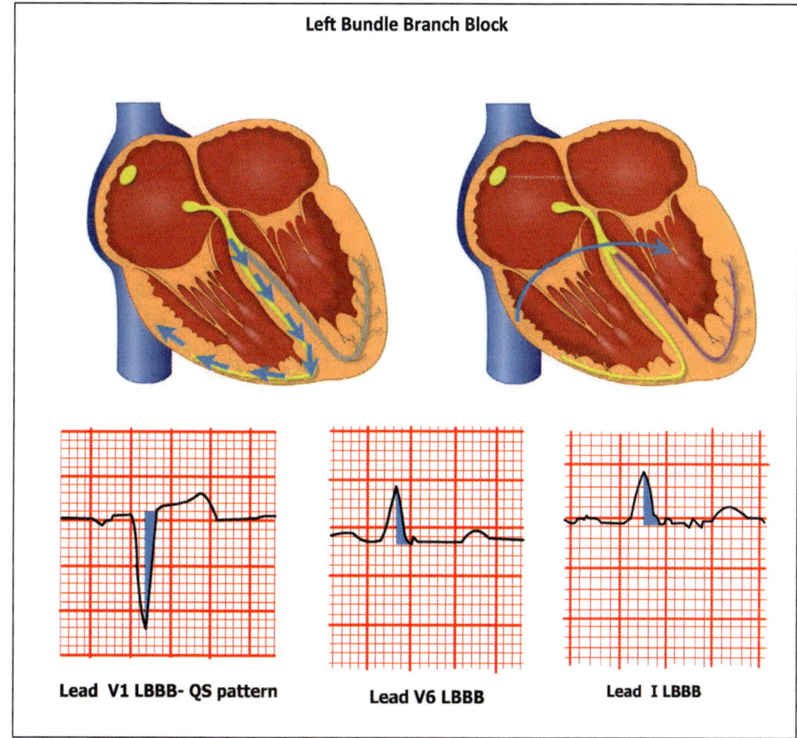

Fig 6.7 Left bundle branch block

and therefore the *last half of QRS direction* is towards patient's **left side and posterior**. (Remember, during assessment of bundle branch block we only look at the *second or last half of QRS complex and its direction*).

- Similar to the right bundle branch block, the direction of T wave is opposite to that of QRS complex in the left bundle block.

- Because of the abnormal formation of QRS, LBBB EKG is *not reliable to measure ischemia*, *infarction*, *hemiblock* or *hypertrophy*.
-

7 Diagnostic Value of EKG

Myocardial Ischemia and Infarction

- **Atherosclerotic heart disease** (**ASHD**) accounts for majority of myocardial ischemia and infarction in adult population.

- Commonly, advanced atherosclerotic heart disease produces a constellation of symptoms known as **Acute Coronary Syndrome** (**ACS**) and **ST elevation myocardial infarction** (**STEMI**).

- The most common myocardial ischemic event that comes across in real world is **Stable Angina Pectoris**, characterized by *chest pain* typically *initiated by exertion* either physical or emotional; which is *relieved with either rest* or *use of nitroglycerin*.

- The characteristics of pain include *squeezing*, *central* or *sub sternal discomfort* (**Levine's sign**) with the *crescendo decrescendo type* (waxing and waning). The pain usually lasts for *2 to 5 min* with *radiation* to *shoulder*, *arm*, *jaw* or *back*.

- Acute coronary syndrome includes two distinct categories of disease process classified based on their presentation, known as **Unstable Angina** (**UA**) and **Non-ST segment elevation**

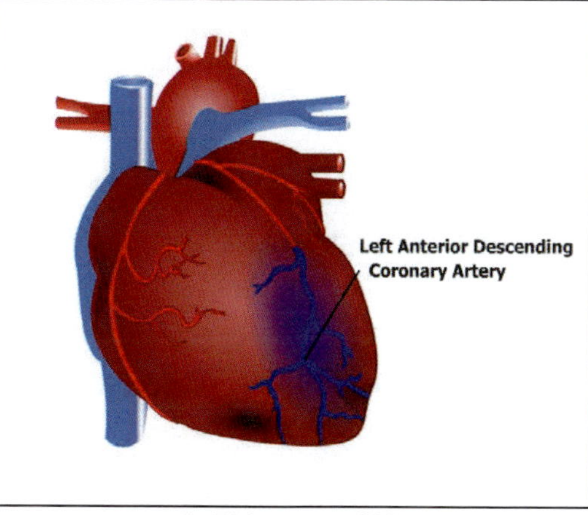

Fig 7.1 Anterior wall MI

myocardial infarction (**NSTEMI**).

- **Unstable angina** (**UA**): Here, the patient presents with *typical cardiac chest pain* with or without radiation to adjacent areas, may or may not *relieve by rest or sublingual nitroglycerin* treatment.

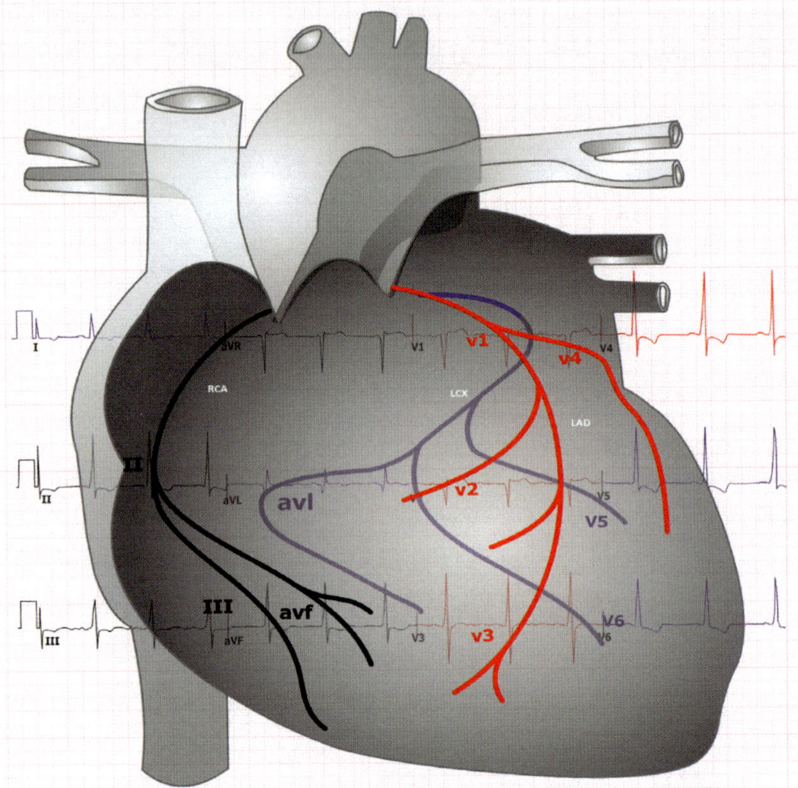

Fig 7.2 Coronary circulation and 12 lead EKG

- These patients may not have any EKG changes or elevation in their target cardiac enzymes such as **Troponin I**, **Creatine phosphokinase** (CK) or **Creatine phosphokinase-cardiac fraction** (CKMB).

- **Non-ST segment elevation myocardial infarction** (**NSTEMI**): In these patients, along with *anginal symptoms* there may be *ST segment depression or T wave inversion* and *has positive cardiac biomarkers* such as troponin I and CKMB. Sometimes ST segment changes are transient (short lasting).

- **ST segment elevation myocardial infarction** (**STEMI**): This acute form of myocardial infarction results from *complete and sudden occlusion of a coronary artery* leading to *acute myocardial injury*. This scenario is characterized by consistent *ST segment elevation greater than 0.1 mV* (larger than one small vertical box in an EKG) in two or more contiguous leads (leads representing adjacent functional areas of the heart such as lead II and III in the case of inferior wall myocardial infarction) in an EKG or *new onset of left bundle branch block* (LBBB) pattern along with angina. There may be coexisting **mirror image changes** in the form of *ST segment depression and T wave inversion* in the areas of EKG opposite to that of ischemia.

Coronary Circulation and 12 Lead EKG

Leads	Anatomical area	Coronary artery
I, aVL, V5, V6	Lateral wall	Circumflex artery
II, III, aVF	Inferior wall	Right coronary artery
V1, V2	Septum	Left anterior descending artery
V3, V4	Anterior wall	Left anterior descending artery

Box 7.1 Coronary circulation and 12 lead EKG

- ST segment changes are consistent with *area of myocardium supplied by the blocked coronary artery*. For example, in anterior wall STEMI the affected vessel is most likely left anterior descending artery (LAD) and is evidenced in an EKG by consistent ST segment elevation in lead **V2**, **V3** and **V4** which are looking at electrical activity on the anterior chest wall.

- There may also be ST segment depression and T wave inversion in inferior leads **II**, **III** and **aVF**, which are on the opposite side of the anterior wall.

- ST segment changes happen because of the *abnormal electrical transmission and subsequent repolarization in chemically unstable environment* that exists in ischemic and infarcted myocardium.

Pathophysiology of ASHD

- The core of atherosclerotic heart disease pathophysiology is a *disparity in supply and demand of myocardial oxygen*.

- Major determinants of **myocardial oxygen demand** (**MVO_2**) are *heart rate*, *myocardial contractility* and *myocardial wall tension*.

- In coronary artery disease, the system lacks flexibility and

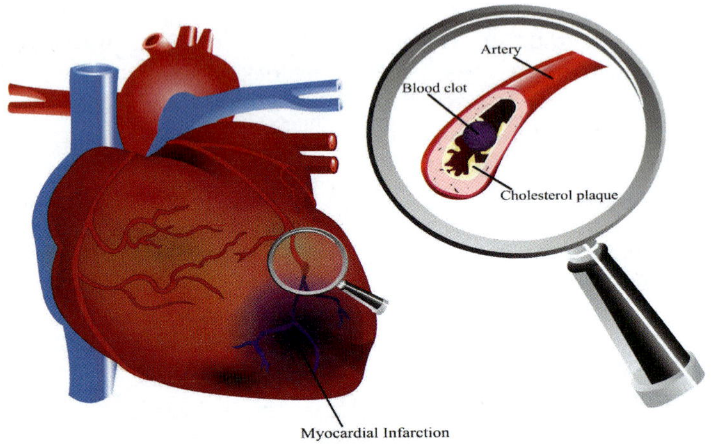

Fig 7.3 Pathophysiology of MI

adaptability for changing needs of the heart.

- Other factors that can adversely affect coronary blood supply are *arterial thrombi*, *coronary vessel spasm*, *emboli* and *severe anemia*.

- Coronary atherosclerosis may be produced by factors such as *increased LDL* (Low density lipoprotein), *low HDL* (High density lipoprotein), *smoking*, *hypertension*, *diabetes mellitus* etc.

- Generally, **50%** reduction in lumen size produces **exercise-induced symptoms** and when it reaches greater than **80%**, patient will have **non-exertional symptoms**.

- If the *ischemia continues for more than 20 min*, *cell death and subsequent scarring of cells (infarction) happens* in the absence of collateral circulation.

- Presence of **Q wave** indicates *myocardial infarction happened more than 24 hours* prior to the presentation.

- **Posterior wall myocardial infarction** is one of the *difficult*

EKG Changes in Myocardial Ischemia

- **Myocardial infarction in progress**

  Elevation of ST segment in leads corresponding to respective coronary artery territory. For example, left anterior descending artery (LAD) occlusion, ST elevation is more pronounced in septal anterior leads, i.e. **V1- V4**.
- **Myocardial ischemia**

  Depression of ST segment with T wave inversion in ischemic territory.
- **Reciprocal changes**

  In an acute myocardial infarction, the area opposite of infarction shows reciprocal changes in ST segment. For example, in anterior wall myocardial infarction, ST segment elevation is seen in lead V1-V4; however inferior leads (lead II, III and aVF) show ST segment depression.

Box 7.2 EKG changes in myocardial ischemia

diagnosis to be made from usual anterior chest wall EKG and is characterized by presence of large R waves in V1 and V2 in a regular EKG.

Events Associated with Myocardium Infarction

- **Anterior MI** : This is the most lethal type of myocardial infarction due to the *involvement of left ventricle and the septum*. This pathologic process can markedly *reduced cardiac output* leading to dreadful consequences if not intervene in a timely fashion.
- **Inferior MI** : This produces *brady arrhythmias and possible heart block*. Since the right coronary artery is the culprit and it supplies right ventricle, patient present with congestive symptoms.
- **Posterior MI** : This is the most difficult type of myocardial infarction in terms of diagnosis. A regular surface EKG with anterior precordial leads doesn't always show presence of posterior MI. *Instead of Q wave, presence of large R waves in V1 and V2 represent posterior MI* (mirror image). It usually originates from occlusion of a dominant circumflex or right coronary artery that supplies posterior wall.

Box 7.3 Events associated with myocardium infarction

Treatment in Myocardial Infarction	
Management of acute phase	Anti-ischemic treatment with • Oxygen • Nitroglycerin • Morphine • Aspirin • Beta-blockers
Preventing progression of acute phase	Anti-thrombolytic treatment with antiplatelets like • Clopidogrel • Prasugrel • Ticlopidine • Eptifibatide • Tirofiban • Abciximab • Heparin
Preventing of progression of risk factors	Risk factor reduction with • Statins and ACE inhibitors • Management of Diabetes, Smoking, life style etc.

Box 7.4 Treatment in myocardial infarction

- Acute management of myocardial infarction depends on the type of MI.
- For STEMI, immediate and timely revascularization, either mechanical (PTCA with or without stents) or chemical (tPA or other thrombolytics) is of supreme priority.

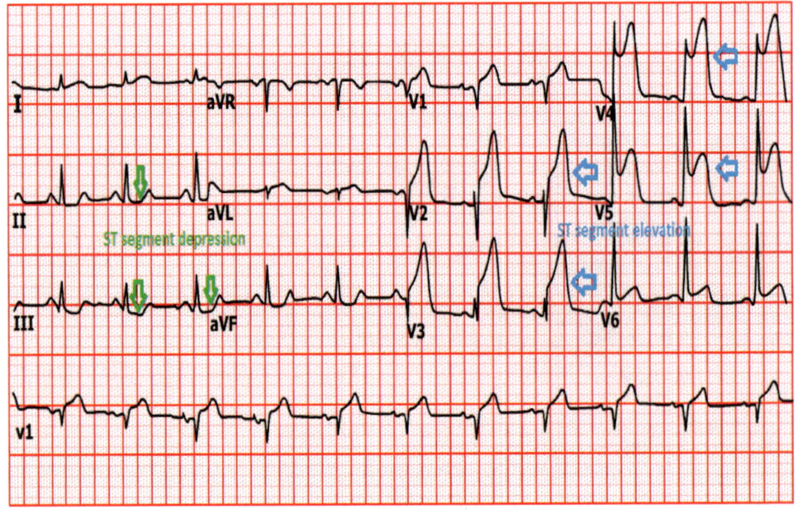

Fig 7.4 Anterior MI

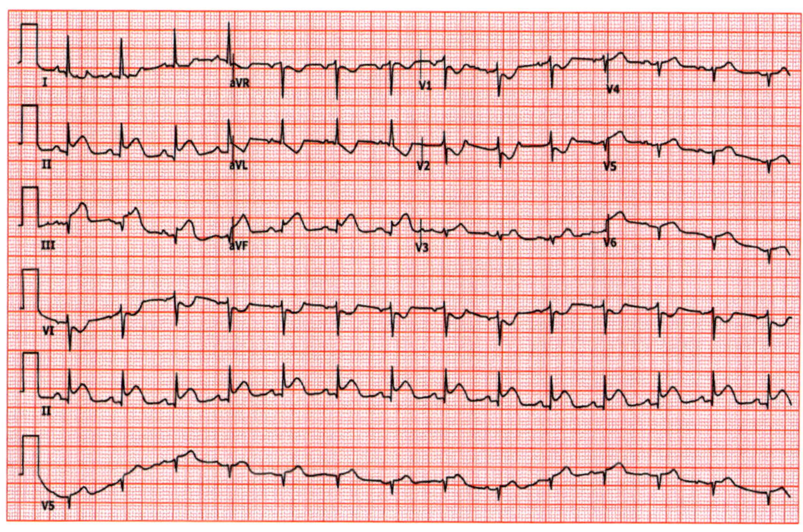

Fig 7.5 Inferior STEMI

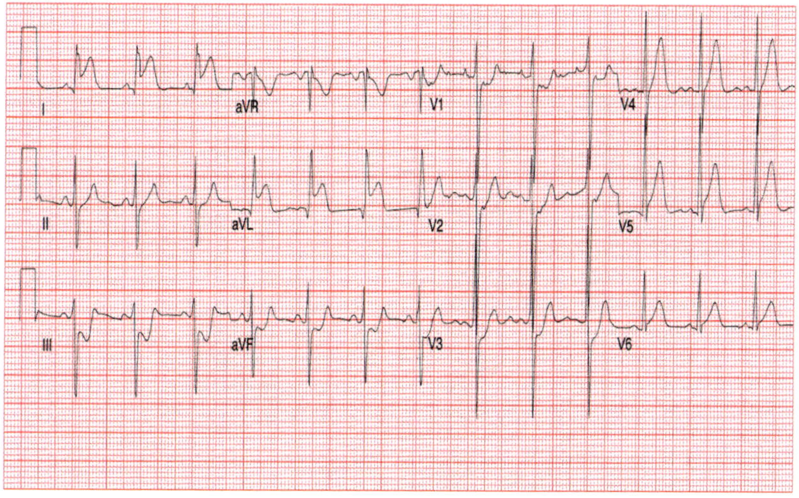

Fig 7.6 Lateral STEMI

- For NSTEMI or unstable angina, non-emergent revascularization along with risk factor modification is the treatment approach.

Left Atrial Hypertrophy (LAH)

- In a normal heart, the sequence of atrial activation starts from right atrium (since the SA node is situated here), which then followed by the left atrium because of the minute travelling delay for impulse from right to left chamber.

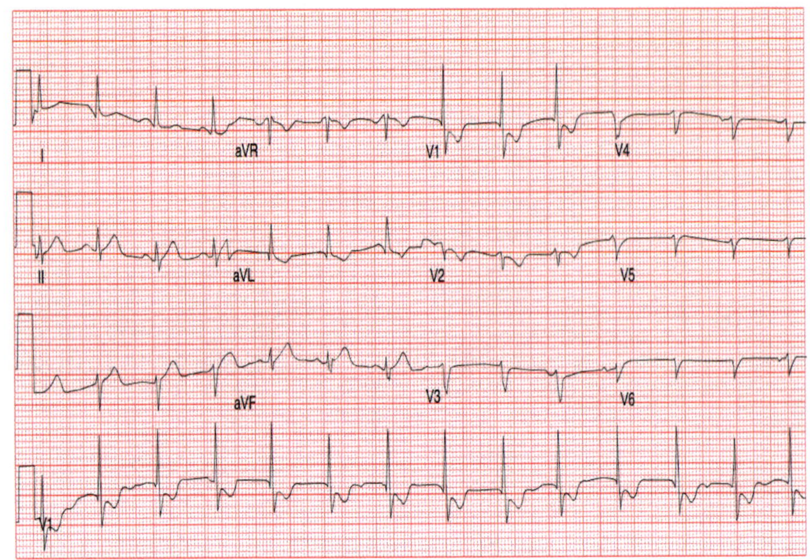

Fig 7.7 Posterior STEMI

- Hypertrophy or scarring of the atrial wall resulting from left atrial enlargement increases this **Inter atrial delay**. This delayed activation of the left atrium leads to a *slight notching of P wave*.

- Similar to any other conduction delay, the impulses from right atrium takes longer to depolarize the enlarged left atrium, leading to **wide P wave** (>0.12 sec) with a **pronounced notching** called ***'P mitrale'*** sign.

- These changes are evident in the inferior leads such as lead **III** and **aVF**. In the anterior precordial lead **V1**; left atrial enlargement may produce a **deeply inverted P wave**.

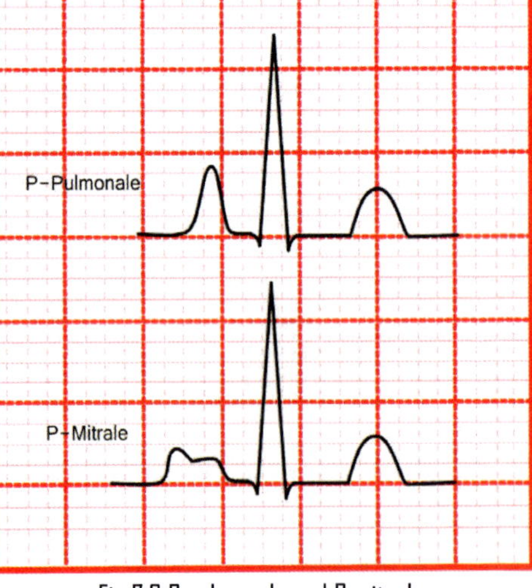

Fig 7.8 P pulmonale and P mitrale

Right Atrial Hypertrophy (RAH)

- Scarring and hypertrophy of right atrium causes *delay in depolarization of right atrium*. Therefore, both atria will depolarize *simultaneously rather than sequentially* creating a *narrow and tall P wave* called '***P Pulmonale***'. This change is pronounced in lead **II** and **V1**.

EKG Criteria for Atrial Enlargement

Right Atrial Hypertrophy

- Narrow and tall P wave (*P Pulmonale*) in lead **II** and **V1**

Left Atrial Hypertrophy

- Wide and notched P wave (>0.12 sec) in Lead **III**, **aVF** (*P Mitrale*)
- Deep inverted P wave in **V1**

Box 7.5 EKG criteria for atrial enlargement

- In severe right atrial enlargement, the right atrium may become so large that it extent towards the left atrium creating an inverted P wave in lead **V1** mimicking EKG change of left atrial enlargement.

Right Ventricular Hypertrophy (RVH)

- Hypertrophy of right ventricle is seen in clinical conditions

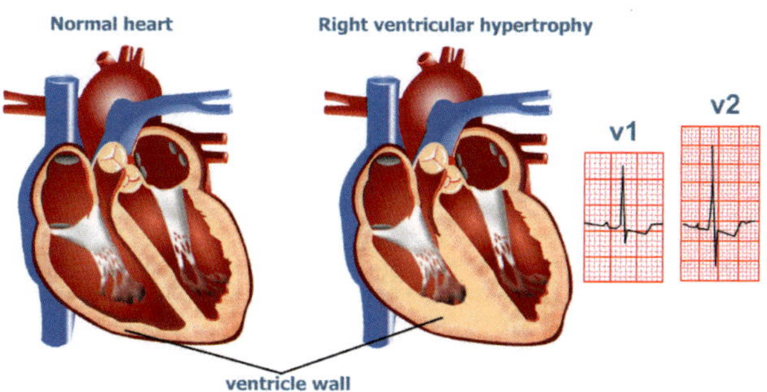

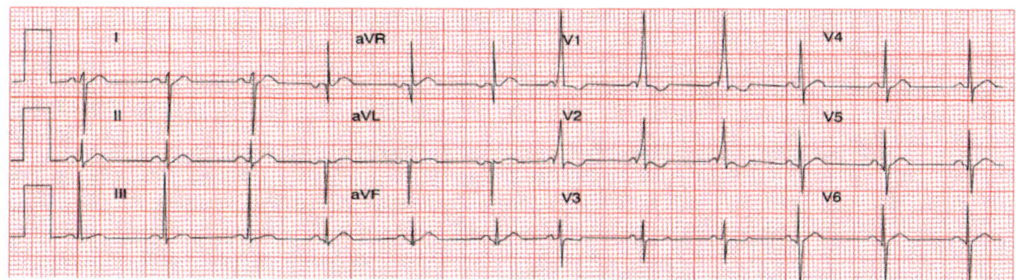

Fig 7.9 Right ventricular hypertrophy

such as *advanced COPD*, *cor pulmonale*, *tricuspid* or *pulmonic stenosis* and as a sequel of *mitral stenosis (due to back flow of blood from left atrium through pulmonary circulation)*.

- This increased muscle mass causes *tall R waves* in *anterior precordial leads- lead **V1** and **V2*** and *deep S waves* in *lead **V5** and **V6***.

- Unlike normal 12 lead EKG, RVH causes *tall R waves and small S waves* in *lead V1* and *V2* creating an **R: S ratio >1**.

- Differential causes of increased R:S ratio such as *posterior wall myocardial infarction*, *WPW syndrome*, *hypertrophic cardiomyopathy* etc. should be excluded before confirming the diagnosis of RVH.

- Excessive thickening of ventricular wall may cause **sub endocardial ischemia** in the right ventricular wall, leading to ST segment and T wave changes in the right-sided precordial leads.

- Right ventricular hypertrophy is also associated with *right axis deviation*.

EKG Criteria for RVH

- Right axis deviation
- Tall **R** waves in **V1** and **V2** (increased R:S ratio)
- Deep **S** waves in **V5** and **V6**
- ST or T wave abnormalities (***strain pattern***) in inferior leads
- signs of right atrial hypertrophy (***P pulmonale***)

Box 7.6 Criteria for right ventricular hypertrophy

Left Ventricular Hypertrophy (LVH)

- Common causes that increase workload of the left ventricle are *aortic stenosis*, *hypertrophic cardiomyopathy*, *long-standing elevated blood pressure* etc.

- The constant strain imparted on the left ventricle results in *increasing muscle mass* and *subsequent thickening* of the ventricular wall. The thickened ventricular wall creates more resistance for electrical impulse to travel; leading to *slightly*

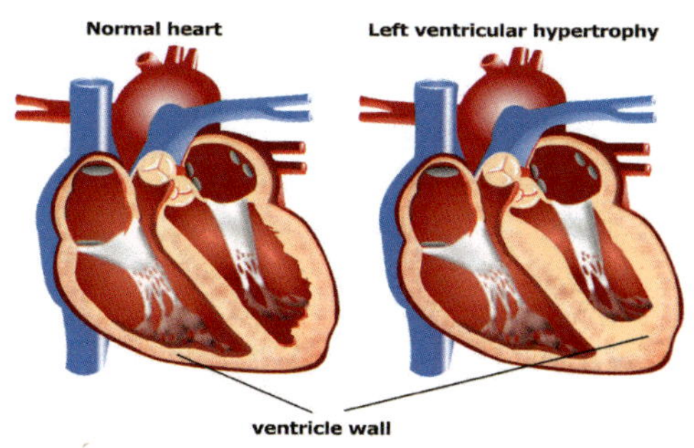

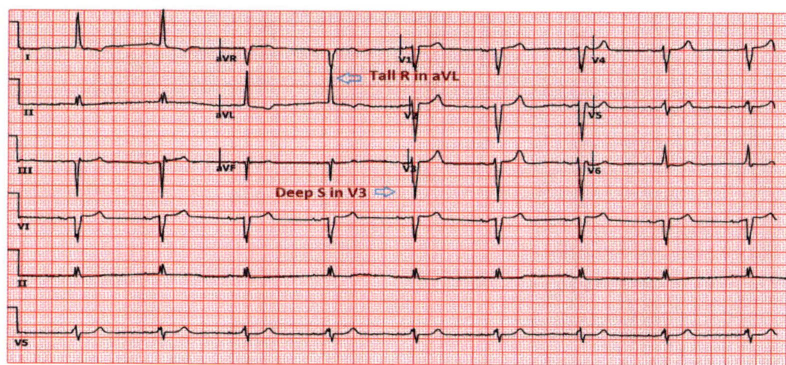

Fig 7.10 Left ventricular hypertrophy

wide QRS complexes.

- Increased muscle mass causes *elevated amplitude* of resulting

EKG Criteria for LVH

Sokolow and Lyon Index

- Amplitude of **S** wave in lead **V1** and **R** wave in lead **V5** or **V6** greater than or equal to 35 mm

SV1 + R V5/V6 ≥ 35mm

R in aVL ≥ 11 mm

Cornell Criteria

- Amplitude of **R** wave in **aVL** and **S** wave in **V3** greater than 28 mm in men or greater than 20mm in women

R aVL + S V3 **> 28 mm in men**

> 20mm in women

Box 7.7 EKG criteria for LVH

waveform. There may be *left axis deviation* because of the increased muscle mass in the left ventricle.

- Similar to the right ventricular hypertrophy, sub endocardial ischemic changes create **down sloping ST segment** and **inverted T wave** (***strain pattern***) in left lateral leads (lead **I**, **aVL**, **V5** and **V6**).

Bi-ventricular Hypertrophy

- These patients may have EKG satisfying voltage criteria for *LVH in the precordial leads* along with *right axis deviation in limb leads* or *tall R waves in precordial V1 and V2*.

Pulmonary Embolism

- Many patients with massive acute pulmonary embolism shows characteristic EKG changes such as a *prominent **S** wave in lead **I**, presence of **Q** wave* and *inverted **T** wave in lead **III***

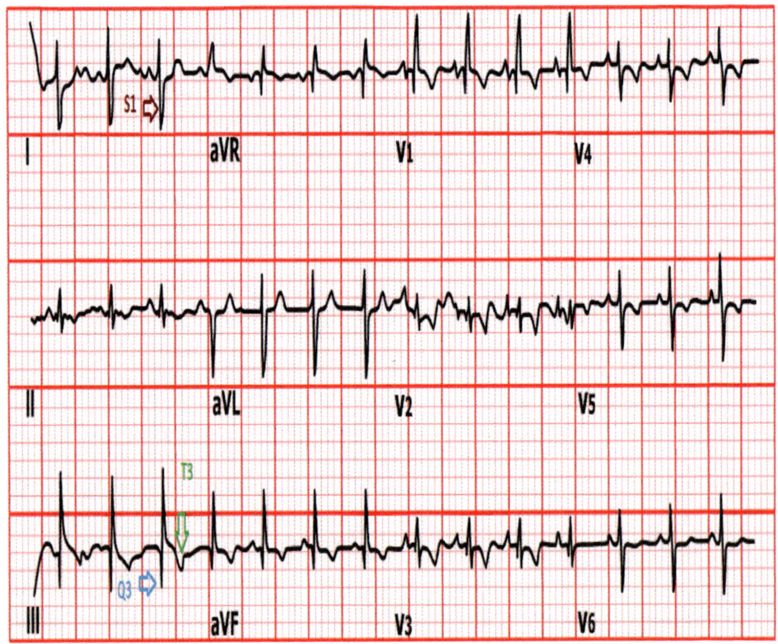

Fig 7.11 Pulmonary embolism

(S1Q3T3 pattern), *ST segment and T wave changes in anterior precordial leads* (right ventricular strain pattern), new *incomplete right bundle branch block* and *sinus tachycardia*.

Pericarditis

- Here, both ST and PR segments deviate in opposite direction leading to *PR segment depression* and *ST segment elevation*.

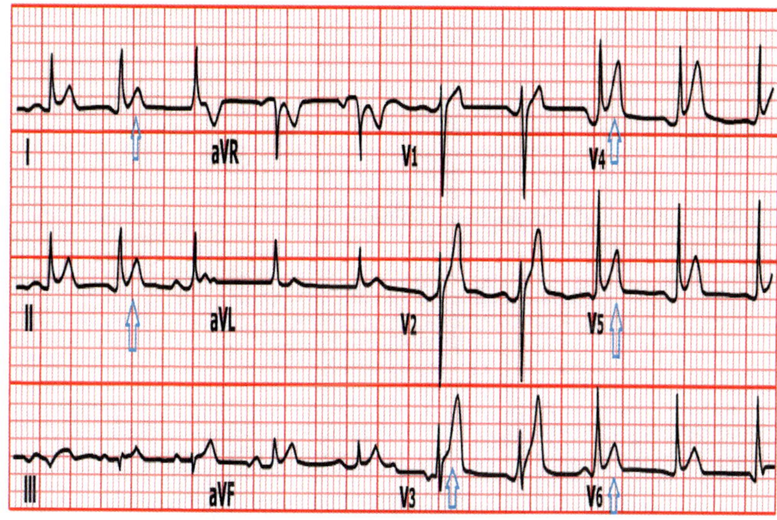

Fig 7.12 Pericarditis

In pericarditis, due to more generalized inflammation and resulting tissue injury, *ST segment elevation may be wide spread in varying degrees in most of the leads* than in selected leads as in STEMI.

- Acute pericarditis can be a reason for pericardial effusion or car-

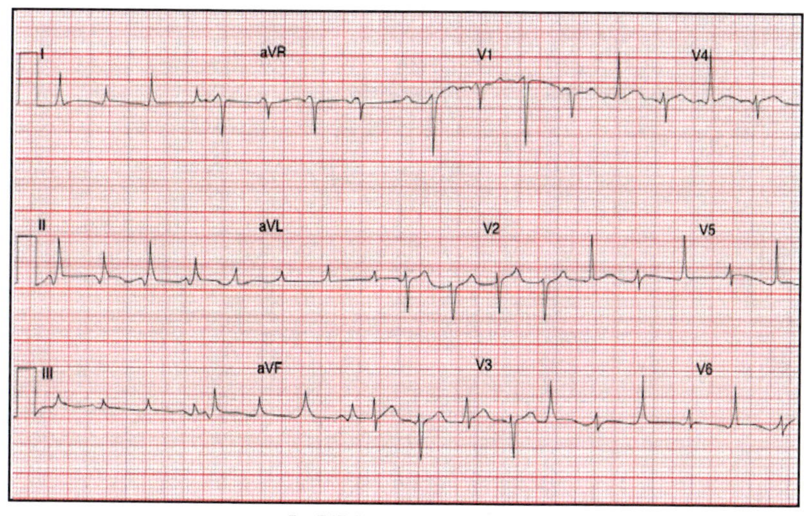

Fig 7.13 Electrical alternance

diac tamponade. In this situation, because of the presence of fluid outside the heart, surface EKG will show *low amplitude or low voltage complexes*. There could also be presence of *alteration in amplitude of QRS in adjacent beats* called **electrical alternance**.

•

EKG Findings in Electrolyte Imbalance

Effects of Electrolyte imbalance in 12 lead EKG

Ion	Hypo-	Hyper-
Calcium	• Prolonged QTc • Flat or inverted T waves • Prolonged ST segments without increased duration of T waves	• Short QTc • PR segment prolongation
Potassium	• Tall U waves • Small T waves • Large P waves • ST depression	**5.5 - 7.5 mEq/L** • Tall peaked T waves • Reversible LAFB or LPFB **7.5 - 10.0 mEq/L** • First degree AV block • Flat/ wide/absent P wave • ST segment depression • Significant bradycardia **> 10.0 mEq/L** • LBBB, RBBB or IVCD • V tach /V fib • Idioventricular rhythm
Sodium	• 'Brugada' like appearance (ST elevation in V1 -V3 with RBBB)	• Shortened QRS duration
Magnesium	• Peak T waves • Prominent U waves • Prolong QRS • ST depression • Ventricular arrhythmia including Torsades de Pointes	• Prolonged PR interval • Increased QRS duration • Increased QT interval • Complete heart block • Cardiac arrest if Mg > 15 mEq/L

LAFB- Left anterior fascicular block; LPFB- left Posterior fascicular block; IVCD- interventricular conduction delay

Box 7.8 Effects of major electrolyte imbalance in EKG

8 Antiarrhythmic Drugs

- These medications are used for management of heart rhythm disorders and are classified into four different groups based on their pharmacodynamics.
- The most common and widely accepted classification is known as **Vaughan Williams classification**. Here, antiarrhythmic agents are grouped based on *their action at various levels of cardiac action potential curve*.
- All of these agents essentially regulate flow of ions to and from the myocytes and thereby manipulate either normal or abnormal conduction pathways.

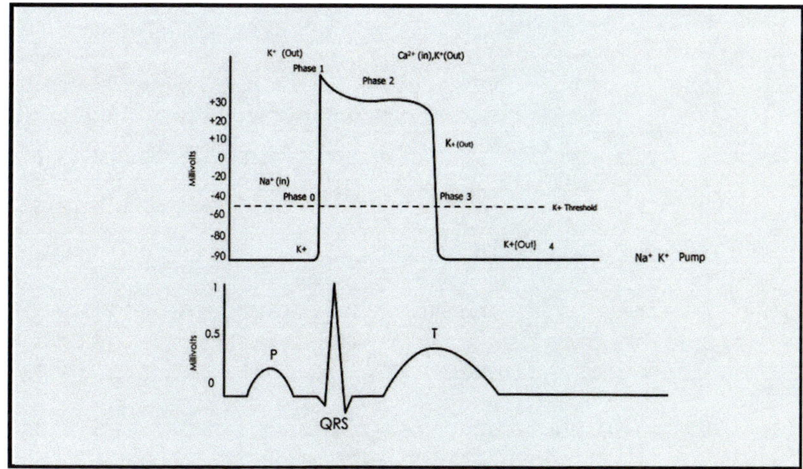

Fig 8.1 Action potential curve

- **Class I** agents are **Sodium channel blockers**, **class II** include **Beta-blockers**, **Potassium channel blockers** in **class III** and **Calcium channel blockers** in **class IV**. **Adenosine** and **Digoxin** are classified as **class V** in this system.

- Even though each drug is categorized in a particular category, their effects may overlap each other.

- In general, *sodium channel blockers slows down the **conduction velocity*** whereas, *potassium channel blockers **decrease excitability***.

Classification of Antiarrhythmic Drugs

Class I	**Sodium Channel blockers**	
	Class I A	• Procainamide • Quinidine • Disopyramide
	Class IB	• Lidocaine • Mexiletine
	Class IC	• Flecainide • Propafenone
Class II	**Beta blockers**	• Carvedilol • Metoprolol
Class III	**Potassium channel blockers**	• Amiodarone • Sotalol • Dronedarone • Ibutilide • Dofetilide
Class IV	**Calcium channel blockers**	• Verapamil • Diltiazem
Class V		• Digoxin • Adenosine • Magnesium sulphate

Box 8.1 Classification of antiarrhythmic drugs

Class I Antiarrhythmics

- These agents are otherwise called **Sodium channel blockers** and they control *movement of sodium ions in phase 0* of cardiac action potential curve.

- By modulating sodium ions at this stage, these drugs can essentially influence the onset of cardiac action potential.

- Depending on the ease of binding and dissociation with the receptor sites, they are further classified into class **1C** (having *slowest rate of binding and dissociation*), class **1A** (with *intermediate binding and dissociation*) and class **1B** (has *rapid binding and release*).

- Because of the fact that these agents vary in their rate of receptor attachment, it is of great use in managing both faster and slower rhythms. For example, **class 1C** drugs (**Flecainide** and **Propafenone**) when used during faster heart rate takes *more time to dissociate from the receptor sites and make less number of receptors available for active contractile function*. This effect essentially lowers the heart rate because of the lack of resources to continue rapid action potential cycles. This property is called **use dependent channel block**. They primarily block sodium channels open for business and thereby slow down conduction.

- These agents may produce pro arrhythmic activity in the myocardium with underlying injury. Therefore, Class IC agents are *not indicated* in patients with *structural heart disease*.

- The efficacy of sodium channel blocking property is *highest for class 1C drugs*, followed by *class 1A* and *class 1B*.

Class 1A

- Sodium channel blocking properties of these agents are *intermediate* to that of other classes of class I antiarrhythmic drugs. **Quinidine**, **Procainamide** and **Disopyramide** are prime examples of this group.

- Pro-arrhythmic effect of these medications can cause formation of **Torsades De Pointes** especially in patients with prolonged base line QT interval and electrolyte abnormalities.

- If the baseline *QTC is greater than 500 ms*, use of antiarrhythmics should be *cautioned*. Therefore in susceptible patients, initiation of these drugs requires *in hospital monitoring*.

- Quinidine is used for treatment of ventricular arrhythmias and Procainamide for atrial fibrillation.

Class 1B

- **Lidocaine** and **Mexiletine** are classified into class **1B** antiarrhythmics. They are particularly *useful in treating ventricular arrhythmias* in the setting of myocardial infarction because of their efficacy *in abnormal myocardium* and also during *rapid heart rate*.

- Lidocaine has extensive **first pass metabolism** in the liver that essentially reduces availability of the drug when taken orally and therefore needs to be administered intravenously.

- Mexiletine is used as an *oral equivalent* of Lidocaine in many situations.
- *Nystagmus* is a common early indication of Lidocaine toxicity.

Class 1C

- **Flecainide** and **Propafenone** are used for treatment of *atrial fibrillation*. In patients *with structural heart disease* such as prior history of myocardial ischemia and infarction, these agents can cause harmful effects and therefore are *contraindicated*.

Class II Antiarrhythmics

- These agents are otherwise known as **Beta-blockers**, with their characteristic beta-adrenergic receptor blockade property.
- Beta-blockers can be broadly classified in to **selective beta I receptor blockers** (cardio selective) or **non-selective beta blockers** (non-cardio selective).
- Beta-2 receptors are seen in vascular, smooth muscle and myocardial cells and therefore *non-selective beta-blockers have global effect* on these target areas.

Classification of Beta-Blockers	
Non selective	• Propranolol • Timolol • Labetalol • Carvedilol • Sotalol* • Pindolol • Bucindolol
Beta -2 Selective	• Metoprolol • Atenolol • Bisoprolol • Esmolol • Betaxolol
* Has more class III antiarrhythmic property	

Box 8.2 Classification of beta-blockers

- Since *beta-1 receptor blockers selectively influence the heart*, they are of great use in clinical situations such as bronchial asthma where beta-2 receptors can cause adverse effects.

- Beta blockers *decrease contractility* (*negative inotropic effect*) and slowing of the heart rate by *reducing automaticity* (*negative chronotropic effect*). These agents are useful in treating both ventricular and atrial arrhythmia especially during high catecholamine states like myocardial ischemia and perioperative stage.

- **Sotalol**, even though a beta-blocker, has *more class III antiarrhythmic* properties.

- Beta-blockers have a wide range of therapeutic usage extending from treatment of stage fright to effective management of supraventricular and ventricular arrhythmias. They are also useful in management of hypertension, congestive heart failure, angina pectoris, hypertrophic obstructive cardiomyopathy, mitral valve prolapse etc.

Class III Antiarrhythmics

- This group of medications have characteristic *potassium channel blocking* properties. Exceptions are **Sotalol**, having *both beta blocking and potassium channel blocking* properties and **Amiodarone** with a wide range of properties extending from *class 1 to 4 effects*.

- These medications are particularly useful in atrial fibrillation, flutter and ventricular tachyarrhythmia. They cause *increase in duration of cardiac action potential* and therefore *prolong QT interval* in EKG.

- When given intravenously during an *acute myocardial event*, **Amiodarone** shows more of *class I* and *IV properties* (*sodium* and *calcium channel blocking*) and thereby effectively *treats faster ventricular arrhythmias*.

- Amiodarone is highly fat-soluble and takes many weeks before reaching a steady state in the body. Because of this extensive fat solubility and distribution, Amiodarone is *not dialyzable* and it stays in body for longer duration. It is predominantly *metabolized through liver*.

- Unlike many other antiarrhythmic drugs such as Sotalol, Procainamide etc., Amiodarone *does not require hospitalization* for initiation because of its low propensity for producing **polymorphic VT** compared to other agents.

- There are many side effects of Amiodarone, mostly from chronic use including **chronic interstitial pneumonitis**,

thyroid dysfunction, **photosensitivity**, **peripheral neuropathy** etc.

- It can also cause bradycardia especially with concomitant use of Beta-blockers. Amiodarone has also shown to increase **defibrillation threshold** (energy required for successful conversion of ventricular tachyarrhythmia) in chronic use.

- Amiodarone has interaction with **Digoxin** and **Coumadin** and therefore requires careful *monitoring and dose adjustments*.

- **Sotalol**, having both beta blocking and potassium channel blocking properties; is widely used for management of *atrial fibrillation* especially in patients *with implantable defibrillator*.

- Unlike Amiodarone, **Sotalol** *reduces the defibrillation threshold*. Side effects of Sotalol include *bradycardia* that is due to beta blocking property and *Q-T prolongation* and *risk of polymorphic VT* (Torsades) as part of potassium channel blocking.

- Because of predominant renal clearance, Sotalol is *not ideal in patients with renal dysfunction*. In patients with risk factors for polymorphic VT (Torsades), initiation of Sotalol should only be done under monitoring in the hospital.

Class IV Antiarrhythmics

- These agents are otherwise known as **Calcium channel blockers**. Depending on the chemical properties and resulting pharmacodynamic effect, Calcium channel blockers are classified into **Dihydropyridine** (**Nifedi*pine***, **Amlodi*pine***, **Felodi*pine***, **Nicardi*pine*** etc.) and **non-dihydropyridine** (**Verapamil** and **Diltiazem**).

- Because of the predominant inhibitory effect on the SA and the AV node, *non-dihydropyridine calcium channel blockers have pertinent electrophysiologic properties* compared to that of dihydropyridines.

- Verapamil and Diltiazem are commonly used for *rate control* especially in atrial arrhythmias. These agents *prolong AV node conduction* and *refractoriness* and thereby reduce ventricular rate in AV nodal re-entry tachycardia.

- Calcium channel blockers can cause bradycardia and especially orthostatic hypotension. These agents are not indicated in pregnancy, post myocardial infarction, severe sinus node dysfunction or conduction disturbance, WPW syndrome, severe aortic stenosis etc.

- Overdose with calcium channel blockers can be treated with administration of **calcium gluconate**.
- In the event of Digoxin toxicity, concomitant use of Verapamil can cause complete heart block.

Class V Antiarrhythmics

- **Digoxin** and **Adenosine** are categorized in this group. Among these, Digoxin implies its antiarrhythmic properties due to *increased vagal tone*. It produces *increasing contractility* (*positive inotropic effect*) in myocardium by *increasing intracellular calcium* concentration.
- Because of the smaller therapeutic window (**0.8** - **1.2** ng/ml), Digoxin needs *frequent monitoring of blood levels*. It also has interaction with many other drugs including Amiodarone, warfarin etc.
- In toxic dosage, Digoxin causes *high-grade atrioventricular block* or *accelerated junctional rhythm* and at times *ventricular tachycardia*.
- In patients with **WPW pattern** EKG, Digoxin administration should be avoided because of the risk of *delaying AV nodal conduction and promoting accessory pathway*; leading to *ventricular tachyarrhythmia*.

Effect of Digoxin on EKG

Digitalis Effect

- Short QT interval
- Down sloping ST depression (Reverse tick mark appearance)
- Decreased T wave amplitude
- Long PR interval

Digoxin Toxicity

Any type of arrhythmia resulting from either a disturbance in impulse formation or conduction except bundle branch block like

- Paroxysmal atrial tachycardia
- Atrial fibrillation with heart block
- Second or third degree heart block
- Accelerated junction rhythm
- Idioventricular rhythm

Box 8.3 Effect of Digoxin in EKG

- **Digoxin immune FAB** antibody therapy can be used in severe digoxin toxicity.

- Tachyarrhythmia secondary to Digoxin toxicity *should not be treated with DC cardioversion* because of the *risk of ventricular tachycardia*.

- **Adenosine** acts through specialized *potassium channels* within the atrium, SA and AV node. Because of the lack of these channels in ventricular myocardium, Adenosine *doesn't have any direct effect on the ventricles*.

- Because of a very short half-life, rapid intravenous injection of Adenosine produces profound and transient AV nodal conduction block and therefore useful in termination of **paroxysmal SVT**.

- If the patient has concomitant use of **Theophylline**, *Adenosine does not work* because of the adenosine receptor blockade from Theophylline.

- Because of the possible micro re-entry circuit within atria, Adenosine can produce *atrial fibrillation in 10-15% of patients*.

- Use of **Dipyridamole** can prolong the effect of Adenosine and therefore should be use with caution.

-

Appendix A

Summary of 12 lead EKG Interpretations			
Rate and Rhythm	• Six second method • Counting small box method • Presence of PQRST and its characteristics • Look for intervals		
Axis	look at lead **I** and **aVF** (*consider entire QRS complex for axis determination*)		
	Vertical axis (Consider Lead **I** and **aVF**)	Normal axis	Lead **I** and **aVF** positive
		Right axis	Lead **I** negative and **aVF** positive
		Left axis	Lead **I** positive and **aVF** negative
	Horizontal axis (Look at **V1**, **V2** and **V5**, **V6**)	Anterior axis	Positive **V1** and **V2**
		Posterior axis	Positive **V5** and **V6**
Bundle branch block	• Look at lead **I**, **V1** and **V6** (*only last half of the QRS complex*) • It require QRS duration > 0.12 sec		
	RBBB	Negative lead **I** and **V6** and positive **V1**	
	LBBB	Negative lead **V1** and positive lead **I** and **V6** (R or R')	
Hemiblock	look at lead **I** and **aVF**		
	Left anterior hemiblock (LAHB)	Left axis deviation	Lead **I** positive and **aVF** negative
		qR complex in the lateral limb leads	Lead **I** and **aVL**
		rS complex in the in inferior leads	Lead **II**, **III** and **aVF**
		Delayed intrinsicoid deflection (time for R wave peak)	In aVL >0.45 seconds
		Do not diagnose LAHB in presence of inferior infarct (prominent **Q** in lead **II**, **III** and **aVF**)	
	Left posterior hemiblock (LPHB)	Right axis deviation	lead **I** negative and **aVF** positive
		rS pattern in lead **I** and **aVL** tall R waves in **II**, **III** and **aVF**	This goes with right axis deviation
		Looks similar to **S1Q3T3** pattern as in pulmonary embolism	
Chamber enlargement	**Right atrial enlargement**	Narrow and tall **P** wave in lead **II** and **V1**	P pulmonale
	Left atrial enlargement	Wide P wave with notching in lead **III**, **aVF** and **V1**	
	Right ventricular hypertrophy	Tall **R** waves in **V1**, **V2** and deep **S** waves in **V5** and **V6**	
		Right axis deviation	Negative lead **I** and positive **aVF**
	Left ventricular hypertrophy	Left axis deviation)	(Positive lead **I** and negative **aVF**
		Down sloping **ST** and inverted **T** wave in lateral leads	LV Strain pattern
		R in **aVL** plus **S** in **V3** > 28 mm in men and >20 mm in	Cornell criteria

Summary of 12 lead EKG Interpretations- Cont...

Ischemia	**ST** segment depression and **T** wave inversion	Lead I, **aVL**, **V5** and **V6**	Lateral wall (Left circumflex artery)
		Lead II, III and **aVF**	Inferior leads (Right coronary artery)
		Lead **V1**, **V2**, **V3** and **V4**	Anterior wall (LAD territory)
Infarction	Acute myocardial infarction	**ST** segment elevation in the target area with **ST** segment depression and **T** wave inversion in the opposite area	Reciprocal changes
	Old myocardial infarction	Presence of large **Q** waves in target areas	At least > 1 mV
Other abnormalities	Pulmonary embolism	Prominent **S** in lead **I**, **Q** wave and inverted **T** wave in lead **III**	S1Q3T3 pattern
		Right ventricular strain pattern	**ST** depression in **V1-V3**
		Sinus tachycardia	
		New incomplete RBBB	
	Hyperkalemia (depending on serum level)	Tall peaked **T** waves	
		ST segment depression	
		Various bundle branch block	
		Severe bradycardia with AV block	
		V tach/V-Fib	
	Pericarditis	**PR** segment depression	
		Generalized **ST** segment elevation	
	Hypocalcaemia	prolonged **QTc**	
		Flat or inverted **T** waves	
		Prolonged **ST** segment without increase in **T** wave duration	
	Hypercalcemia	Short **QTc**	
		PR segment prolongation	
	Hypomagnesaemia	Peak **T** wave	
		Prominent **T** wave	
		prolonged QRS	
		ST segment depression	
		Polymorphic ventricular tachycardia	
	Pericardial effusion or Cardiac tamponade	Low voltage EKG	
		Electrical alternance	Beat to beat change in amplitude

Index

A

B

C

D

E

F

I

J

L

M

N

O

P

Q

R

S

T

U

V

W

Made in the USA
Charleston, SC
18 March 2016